The Vitality Connection

Ten Practical Ways to Optimize Your Health and Reverse the Aging Process

Michael J. Grossman, M.D.
and Jodi L. Jones

Published by VitalityPress Publications

Books from VitalityPress Publications may be purchased for educational, business, or sales promotional use. For information, please write to: Vitality Press Publications, P.O. Box 80903, Rancho Santa Margarita, California 92688-0903, or e-mail inquiry@wanvitality.com, or call 949.770.0723.

The recommendations provided herein are not to be considered medical advice for the prevention, treatment, or cure for any disease or medical condition you may currently have or may develop. As with any change in diet and/or exercise, it is important to seek the advice of a medical doctor.

Printed in the United States of America

*Library of Congress Cataloging-in-Publication Data
is available from the publisher.*
ISBN 0-9727935-5-0

SECOND EDITION

Publishing Consultant: Bud Sperry
Copy Editors: Suzie Franklin DeFazio and Kate Mueller
Book Cover and Interior Design and Layout: Sparrow Advertising & Design
Photographer for Michael Grossman, M.D. and Pauline Taylor, Fitness Model: Hugh Nayeb, Olympiad Portrait Studio
Photographer for Jodi Jones: Donna Reid, dayinyourlifephotography.com

Contents

Appendices

Dedication and Personal Acknowledgments
from Michael J. Grossman, M.D.

This book is dedicated to: My daughters Karun and Lissa who represent my hopes and prayers for the future of humanity; my mother, Bernice Grossman, who inspires me to excellence; my father, George Grossman, of blessed memory, who taught me the living reality of love; my wife, Barbara, who breathes the living reality of love into my life every day.

I have had many teachers who have shaped me in my journey to write this book:

Arnold Foster, D.C., in Brooklyn, New York in the 1970s who taught me acupuncture and herbal approaches to medicine. Jeffrey Bland, Ph.D., and the Functional Medicine Institute have taught me to integrate the latest nutrition research with my daily practice of medicine.

Trish O'Connor taught me to facilitate attitudinal healing groups and showed me a way of being a beneficent presence.

I would like to extend a special acknowledgment: To Deane Shapiro, Ph.D.: For your loving, detailed, and precise feedback on the stress reduction and relationship chapters; your input inspired me to write a more focused and readable book. To my wife, Barbara: For your tireless editing of the whole book and your willingness to refine my first drafts by lovingly thinking out the first three chapters in detail with me. To Jodi Jones: For creating the structure for this project, sharing the process of writing, keeping me on task, and for being a delight to work with.

Dedication and Personal Acknowledgments
from Jodi L. Jones

This book is dedicated to my entire family. To my husband, Dave Jones: Without your unconditional love, support, and patience, I would not be the person I am today; without your encouragement, I would not have had the strength and discipline to write this book. To the loving memory of my mother, Gerry Rado: For teaching me the meaning of giving, grace, and compassion. To my father, Roland Rado: For your wisdom, guidance, and continued support of my many initiatives. To my sister, Leslie Rado: For giving me additional motivation to write this book. To my brother, Scott Rado: For your continued faith in, and support of, my cause. To my in-laws: For your love and acceptance of me, and for your adoption of the many concepts described in this book.

I would like to extend a special acknowledgment to Drs. Michael and Barbara Grossman. To Michael Grossman, M.D.: Thank you for believing in me and trusting my vision. More importantly, thank you for being my mentor, friend, and compassionate preventive medical doctor. I put my health and vitality in your hands. And, to Barbara Grossman, Ph.D.: Thank you for your long nights of loving and careful edits; thank you for making this book one of your special projects. This is a more polished book because of you.

And, to the many wonderful friends and extended family members who have touched my life, for which I am grateful and forever blessed. Thank you for always believing in me and supporting me through this journey. More important, thank you for your compassion and love.

Acknowledgments

We would like to extend our sincere appreciation to the following individuals for their valuable contributions to this book: Kathy Barthrop, Addrian Brooks (public relations consultant), Marty Buford, Lilly Cavanagh, Dwight Griffith, Esq., Jerry Grossman, Karun Grossman, Jacqueline Jacques, N.D., Rich, Lori, and Joe Kemp, Diane Lara (nutritionist), Loriann Lippy, Karen Loomis, Michelle Loomis, Bob and Novene Manley, Jennifer Mogan, Brandi Morinoue, PA-C, Dave and Holly Novosel, Sonny Robinson, Bernie Ryerson, Leon Saunders, M.D., Michael Schleider, Sally Schneider (recipe and catering consultant), Leslie Serrano (makeup artist), Walter Serrano (personal trainer), Deane Shapiro, Ph.D., Robert Shekell, Rod Smith, Jim and Alice Sweet, Pauline Taylor (personal trainer and fitness model in the book), Larie and Katie Trippet, and Hope Witmer.

To Clay Lord, our dear and patient contributing writer: Thank you for giving us the kick-start we needed. You helped make our vision a reality. To our publishing consultant, Bud Sperry: Thank you for keeping us focused, on track, and centered. You've been a blessing. To Heather Buchman, our book designer: Thank you for your creativity and patience. Your style with our concepts was a match made in heaven. To Suzie Franklin DeFazio and Kate Mueller, our copy editors: Thank you for working with us on our tight deadlines. We value your contributions and appreciate your professionalism and sense of urgency.

Introduction One: From a Clinical Perspective

by *Michael J. Grossman, M.D.*

Each of us has gifts to express in this life and in this body. Each of us has obstacles to that expression. We cannot express our divine purpose if our body, relationships, and attitudes are not in harmony. I want to support you to live a creative, authentic, self-expressed life, fulfilling the divine purpose for your being on this earth.

When a tree is ill there are many possible reasons: Bad soil, viral infected leaves, insect infestation, fungal infection, lack of water or too much water, lack of sunlight. When we correct the imbalance then the tree can naturally blossom, bear fruit, and fulfill its function and purpose.

We need to be aware of the connections between our vitality and the balance in our body, our relationships and our attitudes. This includes our lifestyles, stress levels, nutrition, food allergies, intestinal health, cellular toxicity, and level of exercise.

My passion for over twenty-five years has been treating illnesses through integrating natural and traditional approaches to health. While a medical student in 1973, I witnessed a demonstration of the Chinese practice of acupuncture. I was amazed when the upper gums of another student were numbed by a needle placed between his first and second toes. This inspired me to join the pioneering group of medical doctors in 1974 who were licensed to practice acupuncture.

In medical school, I researched the value of meditation in improving hormonal balance in people. In Switzerland and France, I observed that the integration of natural applications with traditional approaches was far more advanced than in the United States. Since my days in medical school, I have committed myself to combine the best from traditional and natural disciplines. Today, many physicians neglect the research on the effectiveness of natural regimens to create health, and they fail to appreciate its importance. The practical applications discussed in this book do not come from abstract research alone, but have been acquired from my twenty-five years of experience in improving my patients' health.

My success rate in treating patients with chronic illness who have seen many other specialists before me has been approximately 80 percent. By applying the principles in this book on a consistent basis, you will feel younger, have more tolerance and enjoyment of exercise, and experience better brain function and improved memory. Patients following this anti-aging program usually feel, act, and score ten years younger on physiological age testing.

I have used nutrition and herbs in my family practice since 1978. In addition to my wellness center, I have taught meditation for twenty-five years, attitudinal healing classes for twelve years, and relationship classes with my wife, Barbara, for twelve years. As an assistant clinical professor at the University of California at Irvine, I have taught nutrition and complementary medicine regularly to medical students and residents. I have partnered with Jodi Jones and the Wellness Alliance

Network for the past couple of years to teach this comprehensive approach to wellness and vitality.

It is extremely gratifying for me to be able to offer specific tools and practical methods to help individuals feel younger, more energetic, and more vital. The most important effect of this book will be the connections you make between your vitality, or lack thereof, and what you do, what you eat, what you think, and what you feel. Twenty-five years of experience has demonstrated that these methods work if you use them.

Vitality is your birthright. After you read this book and make these life-changing connections, you will never again be a victim of diminished vitality. Claim your birthright and make these practical methods a part of your daily life.

Introduction Two: From a Practical Perspective

by Jodi L. Jones

There are dozens of clichés concerning health and happiness. Most people repeat them often without fully embracing their meanings. Until we are faced with a health challenge, it is impossible to truly relate to these simple, yet profound, statements.

"All the money in the world means nothing without your health."

"You don't appreciate your health until you lose it."

"Without your health you have nothing."

I found myself casually using these phrases throughout my twenties and early thirties. Like most young adults, I felt I was invincible. It wasn't until my own personal health was compromised that I fully began to appreciate their true meanings.

Before I share my personal stories, I want to stress that this book is not intended only for people with health problems. It is a book for everyone—especially those invincible "baby boomers" who are now feeling the effects of the lifestyle choices they made in their teens and twenties. It is a book for those who feel healthy today, those who are currently suffering from aging conditions or chronic illnesses, and those who simply want to have more vitality.

Every day, we all experience a degree of health degeneration whether we feel it or not. Every day, we make choices that directly impact our health and vitality. And every day, we have the opportunity to slow down, or even temporarily reverse, the aging process. These opportunities are created by the foods we eat, the attitudes we hold, the toxins we avoid, the energy we burn, the supplements we take—the list goes on and on.

It is within our power to optimize our own health and vitality. Having a genetic predisposition does not necessarily mean you are destined to have a familial illness. Conversely, having a "pure" genetic makeup does not guarantee you freedom from illness. Prevention is paramount. This book connects all the key factors of wellness and prevention to provide you foundational information to help you make informed decisions about your lifestyle choices. Its goal is to provide you with practical applications of some very complex concepts. The choice of when and how to execute them is yours.

As for my inspiration for writing this book, simply put, I am a health ambassador on a mission to reach as many people as possible in hopes of preventing illnesses and optimizing health and vitality. I am a self-proclaimed "prevention pusher."

As a former technology executive who did not pay attention to the warning signs of illness, I learned my lessons the hard way. I fell into the trap of my "Type A" personality. I abused my body by working excessively (or should I say obsessively), eating the wrong foods, getting too little sleep, ignoring stress symptoms, avoiding exercise, and denying the benefits of nutritional supplements. I lived a life counter to the health clichés I mentioned earlier.

The result? I got very sick, took a lot of (toxic) medication, got even sicker, and only then realized I had to drastically change my lifestyle. Within a year of walking the wellness path, I fully recovered. I am a living testimonial to the power of the concepts discussed in this book. I teach these concepts, together with Dr. Grossman and other wellness experts, at our VitalityPlus Workshops to corporations throughout the United States. I also serve as a personal vitality coach to help educate, motivate, and guide individuals on how to transition into a lifestyle of wellness. This formula works; I have witnessed it with hundreds of people. Dr. Grossman has witnessed it with thousands.

I am not a doctor—I am an enlightened and motivated testimonial. My focus is on "practical" wellness. Throughout this book, Dr. Grossman illuminates the clinical perspective of wellness, and I contribute its practical execution. Together, we create a compelling solution for optimized health and vitality that everyone can follow.

As for my personal experiences with various health challenges, I will elaborate on a couple, although I am aware of many relating to other family members and friends as well.

When I was eight years old, my mother was finally diagnosed with multiple sclerosis (MS), after experiencing symptoms since she was pregnant with me. Back in the early 1960s, this was an extremely difficult disease to diagnose; even today with advances in medical technology, it continues to be misdiagnosed. The diagnosis was a relief, proof that her illness was "not in her head" as many doctors had suggested, except for the one osteopathic doctor who began treating her.

Despite her positive attitude and will to live, the progressive disease diminished her health so drastically that she died from pneumonia at the age of forty-nine. Her passing was a blessing, as she had suffered terribly for many, many years. My father, sister, brother, and I were her caretakers. We watched and desperately tried to prevent it as a beautiful, independent, vibrant, and seemingly healthy woman deteriorated before our very eyes. We witnessed the devastation that losing one's health, vitality, and independence can bring.

However, I never realized the impact of my mother's poor health and eventual death on my own well-being. The stress of these circumstances, among others, took a toll on my health. I did not pay attention to the early warning signs and did not take an active interest in learning about prevention and wellness. In my mid-thirties, I was diagnosed with lupus and fibromyalgia, after experiencing symptoms for many years. But I was not the only one affected; my husband was suffering just watching me fight through the pain and constant fatigue. Within a few years, he witnessed his young, vibrant, and invincible twenty-eight-year-old bride slowly transform to a tired, aching, aging woman. Conventional medications were barely effective in treating my symptoms; I certainly was not being healed. I knew there had to be a better way.

Within a week after my fortieth birthday, and within a few weeks of the death of my dearest lifelong friend from cancer, I resigned from my career in technology and began my journey to wellness. I researched the few reputable wellness clinics in the United States. It was during this weeklong series of tests, evaluations, and wellness education that I realized how my lifestyle and dietary choices exacerbated my diseases. I knew then that I had to make significant changes if I was to get better. These changes would not only impact me, but my family as well; I couldn't do it alone.

My husband, Dave, who continued to support me in every way, was cautiously optimistic about this journey; yet he was willing to do whatever it took to get the "old" Jodi back. We strictly followed the nutritional guidelines and the supplementation regimen and continued to learn about the many other aspects of wellness, including stress reduction and detoxification.

Through this process, Dave's hypoglycemia symptoms, which he had experienced for twelve years, were also eliminated. And slowly, the pain and fatigue associated with my lupus and fibromyalgia were mollified as well. In fact, my blood tests today reveal no trace of antinuclear antibodies (one indicator of lupus), and I am completely symptom free. I have my life back and can truly advocate the saying, "Without your health you have nothing."

It is my sincere hope that you will not only read each chapter in this book, but also embrace its concepts and utilize the practical ways to optimize your health and vitality it describes. The power of prevention is in your hands.

How to Use This Book

This is a comprehensive book about health and vitality. The concepts presented here will enable you to execute a practical plan based on your own personal health goals and/or challenges.

We recommend you read this book in its entirety for maximum benefit. However, it is written in such a way that you can refer to only those chapters that address your specific health conditions or areas of interest.

Please note: The recommendations provided herein are not to be considered medical advice for the prevention, treatment, or cure for any disease or medical condition you may currently have or may develop. As with any change in diet and/or exercise, it is important to seek the advice of a medical doctor. Additionally, the information and recommendations provided herein are for your general knowledge and you must take full responsibility for your decisions and actions on any lifestyle changes you make and the consumption of any nutritional supplements.

Furthermore, you release the authors, publisher, and all other companies and individuals associated with the recommended products and/or services from any responsibility and liability associated with any loss, injury, damage, illness, medical condition, or death that may or may not be a direct result from your engaging in the recommended activities or consuming the recommended products. It should also be noted that the FDA has not evaluated or approved any claims supporting the use of supplementation for the diagnosis, prevention, cure, or treatment for any disease.

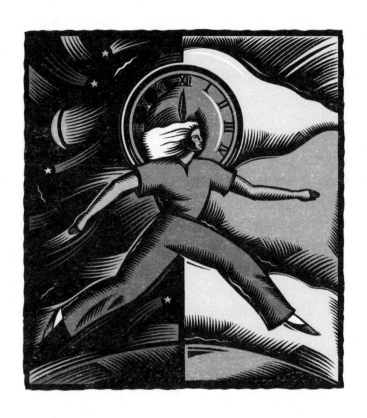

Reversing your physiological age is possible. Inviduals who follow our anti-aging program consistently feel and look younger.

Key Factor One
Participate in an Anti-Aging Program

Scientists are on the cusp of breakthrough discoveries in genetic research on age reversal. We know that the little coverings of our chromosomes, called telomeres, shrink with aging, which activates aging genes. Medical science will find ways to stop this effect and thus truly reverse the aging process and maybe create a thousand-year age spans.

For now, this book is the best information available. You can choose to live with vitality until you are a hundred years old or feel old and sickly at sixty-five. Anti-aging was a part of science fiction twenty-five years ago; now it is a reality.

The prestigious Journal of Science *published an article in May 10, 2002, entitled "Broken Limits to Life Expectancy," which purports there is no limit to life expectancy gains. Until 1950, gains in life expectancy in the United States were due to reductions in the death rate of younger people. Today, the average life span is 76.4 years. If current trends continue, the article estimates female life expectancy to be between 92 and 101.5 years by 2070.*

The recommendations in this book are practical but comprehensive. I am confident that this anti-aging program will not only help you to feel younger, but to live your life with more enjoyment, vitality, and enrichment.

—Michael J. Grossman, M.D.

Premature Aging Assessment

To determine your need for an anti-aging program, answer each of the following questions.

Have you scored your physiological versus chronological age within the past five years?	Yes	No
Has your body fat, muscle strength, or blood pressure improved in the last five to ten years?	Yes	No
Are your risk factors low for cardiovascular disease: Homocysteine, C-Reactive Protein, HDL to LDL cholesterol ratio, fibrinogen, liporprotein(a)?	Yes	No
Are you at your optimal weight?	Yes	No
Are you free of pain and chronic health conditions?	Yes	No
Do you regularly consume four to six small balanced nutritious meals daily?	Yes	No
Do you avoid foods and beverages that contain sugar, caffeine, and carcinogenic ingredients?	Yes	No
Do you avoid fast food restaurants (avoid eating French fries, hamburgers, hot dogs, and pizza)?	Yes	No
Do you exercise for strength and endurance at least three times per week?	Yes	No
Do you take pharmaceutical-grade nutritional supplements daily?	Yes	No
Do you regularly participate in stress reduction practices?	Yes	No
Do you often wake up feeling vibrant and energetic in the morning?	Yes	No
Are your hormonal levels in a youthful range?	Yes	No
Are you taking natural hormonal supplements as needed?	Yes	No
Do you avoid smoking?	Yes	No
Do you avoid alcohol consumption or only consume one glass of wine daily?	Yes	No

Do you avoid sun exposure and use sunscreen regularly?	Yes No
Do you use topical antioxidants to reduce skin aging?	Yes No

If you answered "no" to three or fewer questions above, you have a low to medium risk for premature aging. If you answered "no" to four or more questions above, you have a high risk for premature aging and will benefit by reading this chapter.

Most of us do not think much about our health until the onset of a life-threatening medical condition, such as cancer, or a chronic problem such as arthritis, diabetes, or chronic fatigue, forces us to pay closer attention. By taking an active role in creating optimum health and vitality before serious health problems occur, you can prevent premature aging and premature death while maintaining a higher quality of life throughout your years.

With today's average life expectancy of 76.9 years for men and 79.5 years for women, there are important decisions to make now about establishing healthy lifestyle habits that contribute to quality senior years free of disease, pain, and fatigue.[1]

What you do today will profoundly impact the health and vitality you will have in your later decades. Many people suffer during the last decade or more of their lives as the result of poor nutrition and lifestyle choices.

The Benefits of Putting These Principles into Practice

By incorporating the factors discussed in this book into your life, you can attain optimum levels of health, happiness, and vitality. This book presents time-tested and proven information you need to know to slow the aging process and enjoy a vibrant life. Some of the benefits you can expect to receive when you follow these recommendations include:

- Maximized well-being
- Improved self-esteem
- Increased energy
- A balanced lifestyle
- Reduced stress
- Enhanced job satisfaction
- Strengthened relationships
- Improved quality of life
- Heightened resistance to disease
- Increased brain function

The opportunity to obtain these benefits is determined by your commitment and desire to achieve these results. Your genetic programming is but a small part of your experience of health or illness.

Expressing Your Genes: The Sad Case of the Pima Indians

Dr. Jeffrey Bland, a noted expert on the effects of diet on genes, concludes that, after the age of forty, 75 percent of your health is due to what you have done to and with your genes based on lifestyle and nutrition, not the genes themselves. A tragic case in point is the Pima Indian tribe of the American Southwest.[2] In the first half of the twentieth century, these hardy Native Americans, the Pima Indians, were renowned for their prowess as marathon runners and their ability to survive in difficult situations with minimal nourishment. Their genetic structure is referred to as a "thrifty genotype."[3] The combination of vigorous aerobic exercise and a healthy diet produced an incidence of cardiovascular disease that ranked among the lowest of any group in the United States.

In later decades, the commercialization of the twentieth century caught up with the Pimas. Tribal members abandoned their traditional diet and good health habits and started eating lunch at fast-food restaurants. They replaced complex carbohydrates and high fiber with simple sugars and processed flour. The result is that over 60 percent of the Pima tribe today has Type 2 diabetes; this is the highest rate of diabetes in any one group in the world.

Diabetes and heart disease are epidemic not only with the Pimas. All Americans are threatened by these chronic illnesses as never before. When it comes to assessing the state of general health in America, there is good news and bad news.

Good News and Bad News

The good news, according to C. Everett Koop, former U.S. surgeon general, is that the vast majority of all deaths in the United States are related to our lifestyle choices. Why is this good news? This means you have the power to alter your lifestyle by making healthier choices that reduce your risks for many of the diseases that cause premature death. Here is a list of the seven leading causes of death in the United States, taken from the *National Vital Statistics Report for 2000*:

1. Heart disease (29.52 percent)
2. Cancer (22.95 percent)
3. Stroke (6.90 percent)
4. Lung disease (5.14 percent)
5. Accidents (3.89 percent)
6. Diabetes (2.86 percent)
7. Pneumonia and flu (2.79 percent)

Of the above, only accidents, pneumonia, and influenza are not directly related to poor nutrition and lifestyle. However, pneumonia and influenza are related to a depressed immune system that can result from poor nutrition and increased stress. So in fact, six of the seven leading causes of death are related to nutrition and lifestyle choices we can change.

Even a disease such as cancer, once thought to be caused predominantly by genetic factors, has been shown to be 80 to 90 percent environmentally caused.[4] Most serious diseases and causes of early death are thus preventable and totally under our control.

An alarming trend is that individuals are starting to make unhealthy lifestyle choices very early in life and in greater numbers than before. Genes are not the only inheritance we pass on to our children. Even more important to our health than genetics are the lifestyle choices and eating habits one generation teaches the next.

The following statistics from the 1999 National Center for Health Statistics are staggering:

- 61 percent of adults are overweight or obese.
- 14 percent of adolescents (ages twelve to nineteen) are overweight.
- 13 percent of children (ages six to eleven) are overweight.

The percentage of overweight people (adults, adolescents, and children) has increased an average of 300 percent since the 1960s. Overweight refers to a Body Mass Index (BMI) of 25.0 to 29.9; obesity refers to a BMI greater than or equal to 30.0.

Overweight and obese people are at a very high risk for cardiovascular disease, diabetes, stroke, and other serious health problems. Children are not exempt from this risk. It is critical to take action now to alter your lifestyle so you and your children have an opportunity to lead healthier, more fulfilling lives.

The bad news is that there is now an epidemic increase in diabetes and prediabetes in the United States due to the recent changes in eating patterns (relating to soda, fast foods, and sugar intake) and a lack of exercise.

Physicians report an alarming increase in the number of their patients who exhibit the symptoms of metabolic syndrome or the ominously dubbed "Syndrome X": high blood pressure, obesity, high triglycerides, and elevated insulin levels. It is estimated that 25 percent of Americans display insulin resistance and can be classified as prediabetic.

Ten Practical Ways to Reverse the Aging Process

The following are ten practical ways to minimize aging-related diseases and slow down, or even reverse, the aging process. Follow these recommendations, and you will be setting a course for maximizing physical and mental function throughout your life.

1. Identify a Licensed Health Practitioner

The first step in any anti-aging program is to identify a licensed health practitioner who is familiar with the broad spectrum of anti-aging treatments currently available. You should not embark on an anti-aging program without medical supervision.

The practitioner you select does not necessarily have to be a medical doctor. Many other kinds of practitioners, such as chiropractors, naturopathic doctors, acupuncturists, and osteopaths can successfully point the way and chart your progress. In some states a physician or osteopath, however, may be a necessary health partner in administering the initial lab testing you need, interpreting the results of those tests, and prescribing medicine for treatment of certain conditions.

Breakthrough technology in genetic testing

Decoding the 40,000 genes of the human genome has lead to breakthroughs in preventive medicine. Glimpsing into your future medical risk by testing specific genes is now possible. New methods of testing have reduced the cost of testing specific genomes from several million dollars in the 1970s to about $25 for each test in 2002. Testing involves taking a blood sample or rinsing your mouth to collect the specimen. Currently, testing is available for cardiac risk assessment, osteoporosis risk assessment, and immune risk factors for arthritis and other autoimmune diseases.[5]

The purpose of testing is to alert the individual years before a problem develops to modify nutrition, diet, lifestyle, and toxic exposure as indicated. Also, insights into the best prescription drugs for your particular genetic makeup are obtainable. For example, if you knew you had a high genetic risk for developing heart disease or Alzheimer's disease, you would follow the test results and recommendations of your health practitioner to reduce the risk for these particular problems.

If your current physician is not experienced in the medical supervision of anti-aging treatment programs, there are many physicians who offer anti-aging therapies as part of their practices. The Internet resources in Appendix B include online directories of selected physicians who specialize in anti-aging practices.

2. Score Your Physiological Versus Chronological Age

Everyone ages at a different rate due to varying genetic factors and lifestyles. It is possible for a fifty-year-old man to have the body of a forty-year-old or even the body of a seventy-year-old. If he has the body of a forty-year-old, we can say that forty years is his physiological age, despite the fact that he is fifty years old chronologically.

During middle age, people begin to experience a host of physical and mental impairments, including loss of cardiovascular function, eyesight, hearing, short-term memory, flexibility, strength, elasticity of the skin, lung function, reaction time, and kidney function. A very healthy person aged seventy or older can exhibit loss of mental and physical function to a lesser degree than a fifty-year-old individual who is obese, doesn't exercise, and consumes a poor diet. Licensed practitioners can take measurements and conduct tests to analyze your physiological age. These tests look at the following factors:

- Muscle mass and muscle strength
- Blood pressure
- Body fat and Body Mass Index
- Basal metabolic rate (the rate at which you burn energy)
- Intracellular versus extracellular water (indicates toxicity levels and first sign of failing health)
- Phase angle (indicates cell membrane vitality)
- Waist-to-hip ratio (indicates insulin imbalance)
- Brain function (tests of memory and reaction time)

There are many programs and tools used to assess an individual's physiological age. One highly regarded methodology is the ActualAge Program, created by Dr. Donald L. Hayes. Many nutritionally oriented doctors and chiropractors throughout the United States are licensed to conduct the ActualAge Program (see Appendix B).

It is advisable to continue with regular testing on a monthly basis to monitor your progress in each of these areas. If you are committed to following the recommendations in this book, you should witness your physiological age steadily lowering. Once you are satisfied with your "new" age, continue to follow your healthy lifestyle. It will only be necessary to retest on an annual or semiannual basis.

A major factor in the aging process is insulin resistance and the complications of elevated blood sugar. What do we mean by insulin resistance? Many years of eating large amounts of refined carbohydrates and unbalanced meals can cause your cells to become poor at processing sugar. In response to this sugar overload, your cells will decrease their number of insulin receptors to protect against continued absorption of sugar. Your pancreas will then produce even more insulin in an attempt to overcome the insulin resistance you have developed, which in turn makes matters worse and accelerates the aging process.

How does this situation accelerate the aging process? Insulin resistance causes obesity, high blood pressure, clogging of the arteries, an imbalanced immune system, and general aging of your tissues.[6] This aging process is like flexible rubber becoming hardened and inflexible over time.

A "pot belly" (also known as a large waist-to-hip ratio) could indicate to your spouse that you spend too much time on the sofa with a remote control in your hand. However, to a physician with an anti-aging specialty, it is a clear indicator of insulin resistance and hormonal imbalances due to aging.

ActualAge scoring is very valuable because it points out what you need to focus on for maximum benefit. With the results of ActualAge scoring and precise information about problem areas, you will be on track to slow down the aging process.

3. Evaluate and Treat Your Risk Factors for Cardiovascular Disease

Before you start an anti-aging program, it is wise to be tested to make sure you have not already developed heart disease. Clogging of the arteries can lead to serious consequences, including sudden fatal heart attacks and strokes. If your test scores indicate this is a problem area, the first focus of an anti-aging doctor is to take action to dissolve arterial stiffness and blockage and reduce risk factors for cardiovascular disease.

Cardiovascular Disease Risk Factors and Treatments

It is possible through changes in lifestyle to reverse damage and make coronary plaque regress and become more stable, reducing your likelihood of a sudden coronary event or stroke. Diet and supplementation play a major role in treatment.

Anti-aging doctors use a multifaceted approach to remove inflammation in the cardiovascular system. High doses of certain vitamins and EDTA (ethylene diamine tetraacetic acid), administered orally or intravenously (chelation therapy), can be very helpful in healing damage to the arteries. Taking statin drugs and/or niacin can also reduce inflammation. Certain blood pressure drugs (such as Altace) are also extremely effective.

Research demonstrates that statin drugs (such as Lipitor) can help people live longer. Ironically, their clinical success is not just due to lowering cholesterol. Statin drugs help patients by lowering a blood factor known as C-reactive protein, lowering the levels of oxidized LDL, and reducing the amount of unstable plaque in the arteries. It is important to note that statin drugs are known to lower coenzyme Q10 (CoQ10) levels, an important heart nutrient, and they can have toxic side effects, so caution is advised.

Lipitor is an example of a conventional medication solving an immediate problem by lowering cholesterol, but causing muscle pain and fatigue in a large percentage of patients due to the simultaneous effects of a decrease in CoQ10. CoQ10 must be provided through an oral supplement to make up for this deficiency.

Niacin, or vitamin B_3, is very effective in high doses to decrease cholesterol, increase HDL, and reduce triglycerides. Blood tests must be done to ensure there is no elevation of liver enzymes. Hexaniacinate is a newer form of niacin that does not cause the typical "niacin flush" that often lasts for twenty minutes. Also, hexaniacinate causes less frequent liver irritation than time-release niacin.

The effectiveness of natural remedies in managing cardiovascular risk cannot be overlooked. For example, policosanol, which is derived from beeswax, has been shown in several scientific studies to reduce inflammation, lower total cholesterol, reduce stickiness in the blood, and raise good cholesterol as effectively as statin drugs. Also, a vitamin E derivative called tocotrienol has been very effective in decreasing cholesterol. An extract of red yeast has also been very effective in lowering cholesterol. Patients using any of these prescription and nonprescription drugs need follow-up blood tests to make sure they are effective. Where a natural approach is effective, it often works without causing side effects.

Research has shown that unhealthy cholesterol and triglyceride levels are associated with just over 50 percent of people who experience heart attacks, strokes, and poor circulation in the lower extremities. Almost 50 percent of atherosclerosis result from other risk factors.[7–15]

Additional coronary risk factors—C-Reactive Protein (CRP), lipoprotein(a), fibrinogen, and homocysteine—account for 15 percent of additional atherosclerotic disease. An anti-aging doctor may prescribe a variety of herbs for patients who test positive for high levels of lipoprotein(a) or fibrinogen, including turmeric, botswellia, ginger, and curcumin.

An additional 15 percent of atherosclerotic disease is caused by the newly discovered risk factors of subclasses of HDL (high-density lipoprotein) and VLDL (very low density liproprotein). There are numerous natural and traditional prescriptions to improve these risk factors.

Homocysteine, produced from the amino acid methionine, can be a key factor in atherosclerosis and in artery inflammation. High levels of homocysteine are treated with doses of vitamin B_6, B_{12}, folic acid, and betaine (a beet product), typically for the rest of one's life. (See Appendix C for specific dosage recommendations.) Elevated CRP reflects an increased level of inflammation that has many possible causes.

4. Optimize Nutrition

There is a wide range of foods that individuals can eat and still maintain perfect health. For example, Eskimos can thrive on a staple diet of whale blubber, a substance very high in animal fat. By contrast, tribes in the Amazon jungle can thrive on a diet that is almost exclusively vegetarian and contains almost no meat or animal fats.

The general good health of the Eskimos demonstrates that high levels of fat need not be a problem. Individuals can eat the diet of their ancestors and be completely healthy. What makes indigenous diets so supportive of good health is that tribal members eat foods that are natural to their environment, and their bodies are able to process these foods properly.

Eating the wrong kinds of fats, on the other hand, undermines health. Many Americans have a diet that includes high amounts of hydrogenated fats, fried foods, fast food, and sugar. Eating large amounts of refined sugars and processed foods will not maintain a high degree of wellness. Bad fats and oils can actually be toxic to the body, causing inflammation, irritation, and injury to your heart, joints, and internal organs. Sugar intake produces insulin resistance and contributes to the development of obesity, high blood pressure, and cardiovascular disease.

It is as important to include nutritious foods in your diet as it is to eliminate junk foods. Eating large quantities of fresh and lightly cooked fruits and vegetables is very critical to your wellness and health. You also need to have a lot of variety in your selection of whole foods. Fruits and vegetables contain hundreds of phytonutrients, and you need large amounts of many different kinds of nutrients to be healthy.

A Critical Nutrient for Increased Longevity

You may be surprised to learn that one of the most important nutrients to increase your longevity is fish oil, which contains high levels of omega-3 fatty acids. A myriad of studies show that fish oil helps reduce inflammation, lowers cholesterol slightly, reduces arterial clotting and clogging, and stabilizes the unstable arterial plaque. In addition, fish oil nourishes the brain in a variety of ways.

Nutrition is so critically important to your health and vitality that this book contains three separate chapters related to the subject. Please see the following chapters: Eat Balanced Nutritious Meals, Conduct a Healthy Kitchen Makeover, and Supplement Your Diet with Quality Vitamins and Minerals.

5. Exercise for Strength and Endurance

The difference between an old withered person and a young vigorous person is largely the disparity in their muscle mass. If you can keep your muscle mass high as you age, a lot of things change for the better inside your body, including hormone levels, hormone balance, and insulin resistance. People who retain muscle strength as they age stay younger; and once you lose muscle mass, it is difficult to get it back.

The two types of exercise are aerobic exercise and strength training. Aerobic exercises include running, brisk walking, cycling, and swimming. Strength training or resistance training encompasses such activities as lifting weights, push-ups, and abdominal crunches.

Aerobic exercise is very important for cardiovascular health. One of the most consistent prognostic indicators of cardiovascular mortality is exercise tolerance, or aerobic capacity. Many studies show persons with low levels of aerobic fitness have an independent risk factor for death caused by cardiovascular disease.

Having a stress EKG performed every two years is a good idea after the age of forty. The stress EKG will tell you if heavy exercise is safe for you. Also, it can indicate your risk of heart disease through the evaluation of cardiovascular aerobic capacity, exercise-induced arrhythmia, exertional hypotension, and recovery heart rate.[16,17] These measures obtained using the simple technology of the stress EKG are as predictive as newer, more expensive noninvasive heart testing.

As recently as five years ago, aerobic exercise was thought to be the only kind of exercise necessary. More recent research, however, has made clear that as you age, resistance training such as lifting weights or strength training is very important because of its key role in building and sustaining muscle and bone mass.

Effects on the Cardiovascular System

The heart is a muscle and, like any muscle, exercise strengthens it. With exercise, the heart can produce more powerful contractions and pump the blood through the body more effectively.

Aerobic exercise reduces stress and relaxes the cardiovascular system. Blood pressure can drop from this relaxation, which is more of a hormonal effect rather than a mechanical one. There is clinical evidence to support the idea that exercise produces hormonal benefits. Studies show that when diabetics lose even a small amount of weight, five to ten pounds, they achieve positive changes in hormonal balance and insulin resistance, and their diabetic symptoms improve dramatically.

The benefits of exercise to slow down the aging process are well documented.[18-21] Turn to the separate chapter entitled Commit to an Exercise Program, where you will find ten recommendations on exercise.

6. Enhance Your Diet with Supplements

Every day, our bodies are bombarded by countless toxic molecules known as free radicals. Each cell in your body contains cellular structures called mitochondria that utilize oxygen to convert nutrients into cellular energy. By-products of this process are free radicals, molecules that can attack your cell walls, DNA, enzymes, and mitochondria. Left unchecked, these free radicals cause chain reactions and tiny injuries that multiply into widespread damage and send the aging process into high gear. In addition to free radicals produced in our own bodies, we are exposed to tens of thousands of environmental free radicals on a daily basis. This results in 100,000 free radical hits or wounds on our cellular DNA daily.[22]

How can you reverse the daily impact of these free radicals? The answer lies in consuming food and nutritional supplements high in antioxidants. Antioxidants bind to and neutralize the free radicals at the molecular level, rendering them relatively harmless.

We take issue with conventional medical wisdom and practice concerning nutritional supplementation. Many physicians cling to the erroneous belief that you can get enough nutrients solely from the foods you eat, and that money spent on vitamins and minerals is money wasted. The medical establishment and government nutritionists have set dietary standards for intake of vitamins and minerals, known as Recommended Daily Allowances (RDAs), Daily Values (DVs), and most recently, Recommended Daily Intake (RDI). These standards are adequate when it comes to preventing scurvy and beriberi, but woefully deficient for creating and maintaining optimum levels of health and vitality.

There was a time in human history when men and women could get sufficient quantities of nutrients from their diets. Compounding the problem today, however, is a host of questionable agricultural practices that have decimated the nutritive value of fruits, grains, and vegetables. Widespread use of synthetic fertilizers and the practice of growing the same crop over and over again on the same plot of land, essentially overfarming, have depleted the natural richness of croplands by leaching trace minerals and micronutrients from the soil.

Foods today are less nutritious than ever before. For example, in order to get the iron that was available in one cup of spinach in 1945, you would have to consume sixty-five cups today. An orange that contained 50 mg of natural vitamin C complex in 1950 may now contain as little as 5 mg.

In addition, foods are processed and warehoused for months, which lowers their levels of vitamins and natural antioxidants. Foods are grown to look good and have longer shelf lives, at the cost of nutritional value and even flavor.

It is essential for all of us to take nutritional supplements. Supplements can aid digestion, enhance memory, help prevent cancer, and improve a wide spectrum of physical and mental functions. As with food, it is vital to make sure you are taking the right supplements in a form that can be readily absorbed by the body. In addition, to get the most out of your supplementation program, you must take certain vitamins and minerals together and in the right proportions.

For more details and recommendations, see the chapter on supplementation. Appendix C contains lists of recommended dosages for a wide range of vitamins, minerals, herbs, and other nutrients that will support your anti-aging program.

7. Reduce Stress

Reducing stress is a critical factor in slowing the aging process. Some of our stress is caused by imbalances in our lifestyles—for example, many Americans work more than ten hours a day; others get less than seven hours of sleep each night. Some stress is caused by internal factors, such as our attitudes and beliefs. Other stress is caused by external factors, such as money problems and family difficulties.

Evolutionarily, the stress response had a survival value. Back in the days of our cave-dwelling ancestors, life was a constant battle for survival. Human beings were hunted by a number of formidable predators, and stress reactions actually helped people live to see another day.

When the body is truly in danger and we experience a stress response, it may actually be lifesaving. It is chronic stress, when the body never gets to relax and take a break from a constant release of stress hormones, that can contribute to ill health and premature aging.

It is important to look at the mechanisms that stress activates in the body. Stress produces a "fight or flight" response: blood pressure and cholesterol go up, and the levels of stress hormones, adrenaline and cortisol, rise. The sudden availability of energy resulting from the release of adrenaline makes it possible for a mother to lift a car off her baby, or for a caveman to slay a saber-toothed tiger.

When stress recedes and you calm down, hormone levels should return to normal. Many people, however, are under considerable stress all the time, both at home and at work, so conditions in the body never really go back down to healthy levels. After months of continual stress, your blood pressure is permanently elevated, and your adrenal glands are overworked and never shut down. In addition, this type of ceaseless stress leads to chronic fatigue and blood sugar problems.

Elevated cortisol over a prolonged period imbalances the immune system and greatly increases your risk of contracting diabetes and getting infections. You may also begin to lose adrenal gland function, including the ability to make cortisol, resulting in extreme fatigue and increased inflammation in the body. Your inability to deal with stress physiologically makes you susceptible to all kinds of diseases.

There are many ways to manage stress and overcome its damaging effects. Some of the best ways to reduce stress include relaxation techniques, meditation, exercise, massage therapy, a religious/spiritual worldview, and finding meaning in life. It is also vital to build and nurture loving relationships because healthy relationships are tremendously important to your health and well-being.

One of the most critical areas regarding stress is your relationship with your spouse or significant other, as well as your immediate and extended families. The quality of the spousal relationship is a great predictor of recovery from serious illness and longevity. Studies also show that the degree of closeness and caring that exists between parents and their children can affect the children's health for decades.[23]

We all feel stress, but each person reacts to it differently. It is possible to alter the way you react to stress and change destructive reactions into ones that are more positive and healthful. Scientists can measure reactions to stress by monitoring galvanic skin response (GSR) through electrodes attached to the skin. By using biofeedback and other methods, individuals can train themselves to level out the stress curve.

Whenever stress occurs, we can experience it briefly and move on. Studies show that people who meditate on a regular basis are especially successful at ameliorating the effects of stress. Read the chapter on stress management to learn ten recommendations for achieving success in this area.

8. Detoxify Your Body

At the beginning of the twentieth century, detoxification was a very popular topic in medicine, yet there were far fewer toxic hazards present in the environment. Today, we are faced with a continual increase in artificial chemicals from pollution and heavy metals. Another source of toxins is pesticides; substances such as DDT may never leave the body, and DDT can be passed on from mother to child through breast milk. Tragically, there is little medical attention given today to ridding the body of these toxic substances.

There are many sources through which you can be exposed to highly toxic heavy metals. Daily exposure to heavy metals can be as nearby as your kitchen if you use aluminum cookware and utensils. Mercury is a common toxin that enters the body through diet and dental work. Back when they were put in your mouth, you were probably told that the fillings in your teeth were harmless silver, when they are in fact made from toxic mercury. There are newer amalgams in use today that are safer than those used decades ago.

Fish is one of the most healthful foods you can eat, but it is also full of mercury. Since big fish ingest concentrated heavy metal by eating large quantities of smaller fish within polluted waters, tiny fish such as sardines are the safest to eat. Large fish such as shark, swordfish, and tuna contain higher concentrations of toxins from mercury-laden waters; pound for pound there are thousands more amounts of mercury in larger fish. If you eat fish, which is highly recommended, take 50 mcg of selenium with it, which will bind to the mercury and enable you to excrete it. Also, avoid eating fish with known high mercury risk, such as bluefish.

Toxins travel through the gallbladder, into the bile, and out into the intestinal tract. If your intestinal tract is less than healthy, your body will reabsorb the toxins that you just worked so hard to get rid of, and the process will start all over again. Over time, you will gradually build up ever-increasing levels of toxins. It is essential for you to maintain good intestinal and bowel health to be able to purge toxic by-products and prevent their buildup. For more information on detoxification, refer to the chapter Detoxify Your Body.

9. Receive Natural Hormone Therapy

With age, both men and women have lower levels of testosterone, growth hormone, and DHEA, all critical hormones for longevity and remaining youthful. These hormones affect your whole body; testosterone, for example, is not just a sex hormone. Testosterone maintains muscle strength and keeps your brain and your arteries young. Care must be taken with men taking testosterone supplements as PSA levels may rise, causing a potential increased risk for prostate cancer. Women will also need to address deficiencies of estrogen and progesterone as they get older. Natural forms are best, since the synthetic forms of these hormones may cause a higher risk of cancer. (See Appendix C for recommended natural hormones.)

Hormone replacement therapy is a cornerstone of anti-aging medicine. Aided by a program of hormone therapy, you may be able to choose to be vigorous until you are one hundred, then die gently in your sleep, rather than becoming incapacitated and frail at seventy, then withering away and dying a lingering death at seventy-five or eighty-five. Hormone therapy builds up your body's natural reserves that allow you to fight off disease and damage to vital organs.

Daily growth hormone therapy can take one of two forms: direct replacement of the hormone by injection, or an oral releasing factor that cues your pituitary gland to release growth hormone. Once you are in your forties, you should receive dramatic benefits from growth hormone therapy, increasing your vigor, endurance, brain function, and even the strength and thickness of your skin.

The effects of age on your organs can be dramatic. For example, your skin gets thin and tends to tear much more easily. Your heart, kidneys, brain, and liver actually shrivel up; your reserve disappears, and you become frail. You lose the ability to make new proteins; your body is no longer able to grow and stay firm. The reason elderly people can die from a cold or infection is that they have no reserve with which to fight off even a simple disease that would have presented no problem in their youth.

If you take growth hormone, you can stay vigorous and retain your vitality. Growth hormone stimulates the body to resume cell division and make new cells, rather than just using up the cells you have. When you stop growing new cells, your body lets the old cells die off, compromising physical function throughout the body.

The kidneys offer a good example of organ damage and loss of function through aging. By the time you become elderly, your kidney function is typically one-quarter to one-third of what it was when you were thirty years old. That may be normal for an eighty-year-old, but it means that you will have very little kidney reserve and you will be unable to detoxify your body. Administer growth hormone, however, and you will start to rebuild your organ reserves.

Aging is a process that is, to some extent, preprogrammed in your genes. The genes that govern the aging process have coverings called telomeres. With time, these coverings wear away. When the aging genes are exposed, the body receives its cue to begin aging in earnest.

Someday in the future, humans may be able to regrow their telomeres and cover up the aging genes. When we gain that ability, doctors will not have to give you growth hormones and DHEA; your body will naturally manufacture them, just like it did when you were twenty-five years old. In the absence of that technology, doctors are using natural hormone therapy to reverse the aging process.

10. Apply Skin Therapy Treatments

The same factors that accelerate the aging process throughout your internal systems and organs produce similar effects in your body's largest organ, the skin. Stress, inadequate sleep, free-radical damage, environmental toxins, and poor nutritional habits all take a toll on your skin. Sugar, for example, stiffens collagen and causes skin to wrinkle and lose flexibility. Add the ravages of decades of exposure to the sun, cigarette smoke, and consumption of alcohol, and your skin can really begin to show the damage.

Your skin has a number of built-in repair and replenishment mechanisms that break down as you get older. After about age thirty, oil glands curtail production substantially, contributing to dryness of the skin. Fibroblasts, which generate restorative supplies of collagen and elastin, also lose function with age, leading to sagging skin. The skin gets very thin, particularly after age forty, and becomes susceptible to tearing.

What can be done about age-related skin damage? These days, radical plastic surgery is not the only effective treatment you can receive from a medical professional. Microdermabrasion is a nonsurgical procedure that treats wrinkles, age spots, scars, and fine lines. A skin care technician shoots a jet of fine mineral crystals across the skin, removing dead and damaged skin cells and stimulating the collagen. The technique causes only minor discomfort, is noninvasive, and can produce noticeable results after only one treatment. (See Appendix B for recommended microdermabrasion treatments.)

Additionally, there have been tremendous advances in noninvasive laser surgery techniques that offer lasting results with no pain or discomfort. The newest technique in skin rejuvenation, researched by Christine Lee, M.D., involves using two different laser wavelengths together with microdermabrasion, ultrasound, and topical vitamin C. The Lyra 1064 wavelength laser stimulates collagen growth in the deep layers of the skin that tightens the skin like a mini-face-lift and reduces wrinkles. The Aura 532 wavelength laser stimulates the upper layers of the skin to remove aging and brown-red discolorations and reduce wrinkles. Vitamin C applied with special ultrasonic instruments after microdermabrasion will provide additional rejuvenation for the skin. (See Appendix B for recommended facial rejuvenation centers.)

To improve skin's elasticity, firmness, and protection against free radicals, there is an array of supplements you can take. The following supplements, effective when applied topically, have been proven helpful in reversing skin damage. Look for these ingredients as you shop for skin care lotions, creams, and cleansers:

- **Retin-A and renova** are acidic forms of vitamin A that can fade lines and wrinkles for people with light complexions. People with darker complexions, however, can experience skin discoloration.
- **Alpha-hydroxy and beta-hydroxy acids** are powerful exfoliants and antioxidants and are common ingredients in cleansers and lotions. Regular use can thicken the skin and enhance moisture retention. These may also cause sun sensitivity and should be used in moderation.
- **Vitamin C esters** are a fat-soluble form of vitamin C that can be applied topically. This ingredient helps your body produce collagen, improving skin firmness.
- **Alpha lipoic acid** reduces inflammation, and can produce good results in the battle against lines, wrinkles, undereye puffiness, acne scars, and enlarged pores.
- **DMAE** (Dimethylaminoethanol) helps firm up the muscles underneath sagging skin. Applied topically, DMAE improves the ability of skin cells to expel waste and retain nutrients. Many patients have reported that DMAE tightens skin nearly instantaneously.
- **Tocotrienols,** a form of vitamin E, are powerful antioxidants that can reverse severe dryness and scaliness and provide skin protection.

Skin care treatments are the final component to round out your anti-aging program. Consistently applied, these treatments enable you to have it all. You will not only function at peak performance and feel great, you can also look younger and exude new confidence. It would be worth the investment to schedule monthly appointments with a qualified aesthetician for professional facials. The benefits will be internal as well as external because of the relaxing, soothing experience they offer.

Chapter Summary

Advances in medical knowledge and technology have undergone a quantum leap since the 1980s and 1990s and continue to expand at a very rapid pace. Researchers and physicians have devised many simple strategies to reverse the effects of aging, and medical testing has evolved to the point where the results of anti-aging therapies and treatments can be scientifically measured.

By incorporating the ten recommendations described in this chapter, you can realize significant health benefits. Medical science now offers convincing evidence that following these recommendations can help you feel younger, more vital, more energetic, and slow down or even reverse the aging process.

Ten Practical Ways to Participate in an Anti-Aging Program

1. Identify a licensed health practitioner.
2. Score your physiological versus chronological age.
3. Evaluate and treat your risk factors for cardiovascular disease.
4. Optimize nutrition.
5. Exercise for strength and endurance.
6. Enhance your diet with supplements.
7. Reduce stress.
8. Detoxify your body.
9. Receive natural hormone therapy.
10. Apply skin therapy treatments.

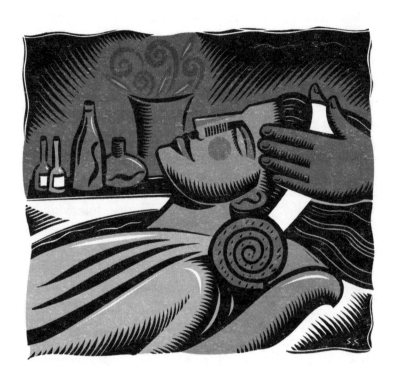

Train your mind to heal your attitude and forever you will feel young.

Key Factor Two
Develop and Execute a Stress Reduction Plan

Stress and anxiety is a problem for everybody. Anxiety was a problem for me when I was competing for the highest grades in order to qualify for medical school. To help me deal effectively with stress, I learned to meditate. After meditating for a few years, I had changed sufficiently to be perceived by my fellow medical students as one of the most relaxed and calm students.

I have had the privilege to teach meditation to more than a thousand persons. The feedback from the positive experiences of many people has been very rewarding. I have also taught classes in attitudinal healing for over twelve years. Every class is a support group for learning to let go of resentments and fears. These groups have been a great learning experience for me while providing the needed support for those who have come to me for help.

Essie, an eighty-three-year-old woman, came to see me. She had been hospitalized repeatedly for chest pain that seemed to be provoked by anxiety. Her children had great difficulty relating to Essie because of her incessant worrying. Six months after learning meditation and attending weekly attitudinal healing group meetings, Essie became much more relaxed and happy; she even returned to her avocation as an artist. She lived another four years, continued her meditation and support group, and never went into the hospital again.

Essie died peacefully at home. I was deeply moved when her children called and thanked me for the transformation of their mom into a loving, calm, and uplifting person.

At any age we can change our experience of life to one of peace and calmness.

—Michael J. Grossman, M.D.

Stress is not avoidable, but it is manageable. We all experience many events in our lives that create stress. Whether consciously or unconsciously, we react to situations that produce fear, anger, frustration, and uncertainty, and this leads us to harmful physiological and emotional results. Unless redirected in some positive way, chronic stress will have a detrimental impact, ranging from mild to serious, on our overall health and well-being.

Scientific research has established a link between stress and cardiovascular disease, arthritis, gastrointestinal and neurological disorders, anxiety, and depression, as well as a connection with many immune system disorders from cancer to the common cold. Overstressed people are also more commonly afflicted by sleep disorders, tension and migraine headaches, and acid indigestion.

Fortunately, prominent physicians, psychologists, and psychoneuroimmunologists have been evaluating the causes and effects of stress for many decades. These specialists offer simple diagnostic tools to help you evaluate your current level of stress. They also recommend tools to manage your stress. In this chapter we will look at the kind of stress in your life and how you respond to that stress.

In Neanderthal days, getting a jolt of adrenaline was probably just what you needed to prepare for battle with a saber-toothed tiger. Today, however, something relatively trivial may elicit the release of adrenaline, such as someone cutting you off on the freeway or a slow cashier at the grocery store when you are in a rush.

In the brain, the hypothalamus releases hormones that initiate the stress response throughout the body. Cortisol is a stress response hormone released from the adrenal glands. Excessive release of cortisol causes a cascade of changes in the body's physiology. This can cause damage to white blood cells, which are vital to the immune system. Sex hormones are reduced, which reduces libido and creates menstrual problems. The digestive tract shuts down, resulting in bloating, nausea, cramps, and diarrhea. Sugar is released in the bloodstream, increasing the likelihood of diabetes over time. Cholesterol increases, promoting heart disease. Heart rate and blood pressure increase, and blood thickens and coagulates more easily to prevent bleeding, leading to stroke and heart attack.

Many studies have demonstrated strong correlations between stress and illness:

- **Allergies and asthma** have been associated with emotional factors of anxiety and conflict.[1,2]
- **Heart disease** is related to feelings of hostility, anger, cynical mistrust, and social isolation.[3-8]
- **Arthritis** is linked to helplessness, trying to be nice and holding in anger.[9-11]
- **Backaches** have been tied to emotional upsets.

- **Cancer** studies suggest that responding to stress with hopelessness and repressing unpleasant emotions can promote this disease.[12,13]
- **Diabetes** can be exacerbated by stress and anxiety.[14]
- **High blood pressure** is related to anger, hostility, difficult interpersonal relationships, and repression of emotions.[15]
- **Irritable bowel syndrome** has been linked to worrying, anxiety, and depression.[16]
- **Frequent infections** are caused by decreased immune function and linked to psychological stress and sleep deprivation. [17]

When you experience negative emotions, there is a specific physiological and chemical correlate in the body and in the brain. Living in a frequent state of negative emotions and subsequent chemical imbalances is very detrimental to your body and your health. Continual stress can create many of the conditions that lead to serious illness. We can experience the increase of stress in the following four stages:

Stage 1: Full energy

Good health means no fatigue; life is a creative challenge and there is enthusiasm and energy all day to meet the challenges of life.

Stage 2: Mild fatigue

Stress initially appears as a minor imbalance in your mind and body. Ongoing stress slowly reduces your maximum effectiveness. You feel tired at the end of the workday; however, in the morning, you feel rejuvenated.

Stage 3: Moderate fatigue

As stress continues to mount, you become tired before the day's work is over. You need coffee and other stimulants to keep you going through the day. By the end of the workday, you are extremely tired. After a night's sleep, you are often still tired.

Stage 4: Extreme fatigue

Over time, with continued stress, you feel overwhelmed and exhausted. You have difficulty concentrating. You are emotionally unstable. You get no relief from a night's sleep.

Resolving the Stress in Your Life

To reverse the debilitating effects of chronic stress, you need an effective plan to restore your balance and well-being. Effective stress reduction requires you to identify and reflect on problem areas in your life. You may need to learn how to think differently about challenges and change how your body responds physiologically to stressful events. You will need to explore various tools and techniques for managing stress to determine what kind of strategies work best for you.

The ten recommendations in this chapter focus on assessing the symptoms of stress you are experiencing, and the sources of stress in your life. Once you have completed the assessment process, you can develop and then execute a workable stress reduction plan.

Ten Practical Ways to Reduce Stress

1. Identify your current signs and symptoms of stress.

The first step to ridding yourself of the effects of stress is to become aware of how stress is manifesting itself in your mind, body, and emotions. Researchers at the University of Miami have compiled a list of stress symptoms and grouped them into five categories: cognitive, emotional, behavioral, physiological, and social.[18] Complete the self-assessment below to gain an understanding of how stress may be affecting you in each of these five areas.

Scoring Key. Circle the number that best describes your response to each statement.

1 = never
2 = rarely
3 = sometimes
4 = often
5 = constantly

Cognitive Symptoms

I have anxious thoughts.	1	2	3	4	5
I have fearful thoughts.	1	2	3	4	5
I have angry thoughts.	1	2	3	4	5
I have hopeless thoughts.	1	2	3	4	5
I have poor concentration and memory.	1	2	3	4	5

Emotional Symptoms

I feel tense and easily agitated.	1	2	3	4	5
I feel nervous and jittery.	1	2	3	4	5
I feel irritable.	1	2	3	4	5
I feel hostile.	1	2	3	4	5
I feel restless or worried.	1	2	3	4	5
I have frightening dreams that wake me up.	1	2	3	4	5
I feel depressed or sad or blue.	1	2	3	4	5

Behavioral Symptoms

I avoid tasks.	1	2	3	4	5
I have difficulty completing work assignments.	1	2	3	4	5
I sleep poorly.	1	2	3	4	5
I cannot sit still.	1	2	3	4	5
I am experiencing tremors.	1	2	3	4	5

I am experiencing clenching of my fists or jaw.	1	2	3	4	5
I cry for little reason.	1	2	3	4	5
I am experiencing an increase or decrease in my appetite.	1	2	3	4	5
I am smoking more.	1	2	3	4	5
I am drinking too much alcohol.	1	2	3	4	5

Physiological Symptoms

The muscles in my neck, back, or shoulders are stiff or tense.	1	2	3	4	5
I am grinding my teeth or experiencing jaw pain.	1	2	3	4	5
I have tension headaches.	1	2	3	4	5
I experience hyperventilation (shortness of breath), a choking feeling, or difficulty in swallowing.	1	2	3	4	5
I am experiencing twitching in my face or other areas.	1	2	3	4	5
I have frequent stomachaches or diarrhea.	1	2	3	4	5
I am experiencing fatigue or shakiness.	1	2	3	4	5
My heartbeat seems loud, strong, or uncomfortable.	1	2	3	4	5
I crave salt or salty foods.	1	2	3	4	5

Social Symptoms

I feel withdrawn from others.	1	2	3	4	5
People bother me.	1	2	3	4	5
I feel uncomfortable when I am alone.	1	2	3	4	5

It is common for most people, even those who would not describe themselves as stressed, to exhibit some of the above symptoms. By assessing the symptoms you are currently experiencing, you have identified possible areas of concern.

- **A few scores of 3** suggest that stress is accumulating in your life.
- **Many scores of 3** suggest you are probably in the mild fatigue stage.
- **Scores in the 4 or 5 range** suggest you are in the moderate fatigue stage or extreme fatigue stage.

You will be able to address causes of your symptoms when you develop your personal stress reduction plan later in this chapter.

2. Identify external life events that may be causing you stress.

Stress experts draw a clear distinction between internal and external sources of stress. Following is a test called the Social Readjustment Rating Scale, by Holmes and Rahe, which is among the most commonly used clinical tools for rating an individual's stress level based on conscious stressful events. Holmes and Rahe studied different life crises and events, and assigned a number of points called "Life Crisis Units" (LCUs) to each based on how much stress the event produces. This scale was first published in 1967 in the *Journal of Psychosomatic Research*. It is as relevant today as it was then.

Take this test now to determine how much potential stress from external events is present in your life.

Holmes and Rahe Life Crisis Scoring Table

Event (occurring in the past year)	Points (LCUs)
☐ Death of spouse	100
☐ Divorce	73
☐ Separation	65
☐ Jail term	63
☐ Death of close family member	63
☐ Personal illness or injury	53
☐ Marriage	50
☐ Fired at work	47
☐ Marital reconciliation	45
☐ Retirement	45
☐ Change in health of family member	44
☐ Pregnancy	40
☐ Sex difficulties	39
☐ Gain of new family member	39
☐ Business readjustment	38
☐ Change in financial state	38
☐ Death of close friend	37
☐ Change to a different line of work	36
☐ Change in number of arguments with spouse	35
☐ A large mortgage or loan	30
☐ Foreclosure of mortgage or loan	30
☐ Change in responsibilities at work	29
☐ Son or daughter leaving home	29
☐ Trouble with in-laws	29
☐ Outstanding personal achievement	28
☐ Spouse begins or stops work	26
☐ Begin or end of school or college	26
☐ Change in living conditions	25

☐ Change in personal habits	24
☐ Trouble with boss	23
☐ Change in work hours or conditions	20
☐ Change in residence	20
☐ Change in school or college	20
☐ Change in recreation	19
☐ Change in church activities	19
☐ Change in social activities	18
☐ A moderate loan or mortgage	17
☐ Change in sleeping habits	16
☐ Change in number of family get-togethers	15
☐ Change in eating habits	15
☐ Holiday	13
☐ Christmas	12
☐ Minor violations of law	11

TOTAL POINTS _____

SCORING TABLE

Scoring	Probability of Serious Illness
Average Person	30 percent
150–199	37 percent
200–299	50 percent
300 and over	80 percent

According to this table, the probability that an average person will become seriously ill in the next year is about 30 percent. High scores on the above test can raise your probability to 50 or even 80 percent. Even if your score is high, however, you can avoid health risks if you take steps now to manage your stress.

This questionnaire also points out how health risks mount when you experience multiple life crises in a short span of time. If you just broke up with your fiancé, it may not be the best time to quit your job or to stop smoking. If you know that you will shortly be making a lot of changes in your life and thereby elevating your stress level, you can best prepare yourself by implementing a stress reduction plan today.

As critical as these profound life events may be as a source of stress, researchers have found that the majority of stress is a result of unconscious factors, stress in our lives about which we are not consciously aware.

3. Identify your internal sources of stress.

You can experience significant stress without going through a life crisis that is beyond your control. Some sources of stress are subtle, such as a lack of meaning in your job, or imbalances in your daily routine that create stressful time pressures.

Beliefs, attitudes, and emotions also play a part in stress. Simple negativity can confer a full range of stress-related symptoms; conversely, a positive attitude can give you some measure of immunity against the effects of stress.

According to stress researcher Suzanne Kobasa, Ph.D., people who handle stress well share the following three traits:[19]

1. A commitment to important values, including family, work, and self.
2. A sense of personal control of one's life.

3. The viewpoint that change is a challenge.

Dr. Kobasa's findings regarding values, control, and challenge are reflected in our assessment that follows. Complete this questionnaire to increase your awareness of the stress you may be experiencing from more subtle sources.

Scoring Key. Circle the number that best describes your response to each statement.

1 = agree strongly
2 = agree
3 = not sure
4 = disagree
5 = disagree strongly

Some questions have an "A" next to them. We are suggesting here that a score of 3 or more on these questions requires some letting go or acceptance. Questions with an "M" next to them suggest that mastery or new skills are required. Questions with an "A,M" may require both letting go and mastery of a skill.

SOURCES OF STRESS

Financial

I usually do not worry about finances.	A,M	1	2	3	4	5
I have a budget plan that works for me.	M	1	2	3	4	5
I can usually save money every month.	M	1	2	3	4	5
I am envious of people with more money than I have.	A,M	1	2	3	4	5

Job/Career

I like my job/career.	A,M	1	2	3	4	5
When I give my best effort at work, it makes a difference.	M	1	2	3	4	5
When I have nothing to do at work, I am uncomfortable.	M	1	2	3	4	5

My job has meaning and I am committed to it.	M	1	2	3	4	5
I get along well with others at work.	A,M	1	2	3	4	5
I rarely feel overwhelmed by the demands of my job.	A,M	1	2	3	4	5

Relationships

I am in a happy marriage or satisfying long-term commitment. (If under twenty-five years old: I love and respect my parents.)	A,M	1	2	3	4	5
I do not hold grudges or resentments against others.	A	1	2	3	4	5
I enjoy my family.	A,M	1	2	3	4	5
I can hear out another person's point of view without interrupting.	A	1	2	3	4	5
I make and keep close friends.	A,M	1	2	3	4	5

Daily Routines

I have a regular daily routine.	M	1	2	3	4	5
I have a regular work routine.	M	1	2	3	4	5
I generally do not feel rushed during the day.	A,M	1	2	3	4	5
I complete the tasks that need to get done.	A,M	1	2	3	4	5
I fall asleep easily and sleep enough hours.	A,M	1	2	3	4	5

Spiritual

I feel that I am a part of a religious/spiritual community.	A,M	1	2	3	4	5
I read something spiritually uplifting on a regular basis.	A,M	1	2	3	4	5
My spiritual beliefs are a source of encouragement.	A,M	1	2	3	4	5

Physiological/Health

I am rarely tired during the day.	A,M	1	2	3	4	5
I know how to relax my mind and body without medication or alcohol.	A,M	1	2	3	4	5
I wake up refreshed in the morning.	A,M	1	2	3	4	5
I rarely get colds.	A,M	1	2	3	4	5
I exercise at least three times per week.	A,M	1	2	3	4	5

Beliefs and Attitudes

I don't get upset with people in order to control them.	A	1	2	3	4	5
I have forgiven anyone who has ever hurt me.	A	1	2	3	4	5
Upon awakening, I am eager to start the day.	A,M	1	2	3	4	5
Luck is not important to my success.	M	1	2	3	4	5
I vote in almost every election.	M	1	2	3	4	5
When I get close to people, I can still say no to requests.	M	1	2	3	4	5
The quality of my relationships seems rarely to be determined by fate.	M	1	2	3	4	5
I would be willing to work for 30 percent less money if I found the job really fulfilling.	M	1	2	3	4	5
I think of myself as free to choose what I do in life.	M	1	2	3	4	5
I would rather be happy than be right.	A	1	2	3	4	5
Finding new challenges in life is important to me.	A,M	1	2	3	4	5

Emotions and Feelings

I am not made nervous by being with nervous people.	A,M	1	2	3	4	5
I am a happy person.	A,M	1	2	3	4	5

I rarely get upset.	A	1	2	3	4	5
If I get upset, it goes away quickly.	A	1	2	3	4	5
I rarely think of past events that continue to make me unhappy.	A	1	2	3	4	5
I am able to give and receive love easily and comfortably.	A	1	2	3	4	5

Scores of 3 suggest that you need to think about that area closely as it may be a source of stress. Scores of 4 or 5 suggest that you have work to do to change things that build stress in your life.

4. Carefully examine the results of the stress assessment tests you completed thus far to determine areas in which you could improve your skills of mastery and acceptance.

Now that you have identified your areas of stress, you can consider possible solutions. The first step is to determine whether your stress is caused by issues that are within your control, or situations beyond your control.

If the stress is coming from negative or faulty attitudes and beliefs, learn how to change your attitudes and beliefs. If the stress is from factors outside your control, you need to learn to let go and accept what is. If the stress is due to lack of skills, this may be the time to gain mastery in that area.

A sense of control is a very important part of psychological and physical health. Healthy control can be achieved in one of two ways: by letting go and gaining acceptance of life situations, or by acting with mastery to solve problems and create good results.

By trying to take charge of situations that are out of your control, you can create stress that leads to heart disease, high blood pressure, or stomach ulcers. Feeling the aggressive emotions of anger, indignation, resentment, irritation, and impatience are signs of overcontrol. If you find that you would rather be right than be happy, your style probably can be characterized as overcontrolling.

In contrast, feelings of helplessness or hopelessness are associated with low-functioning immune system diseases, such as cancer and arthritis. People who feel helpless or hopeless do not act on problems that are within their control; they are overly submissive, do not express themselves freely, and choose not to say and do things that could improve their situation. This style can be characterized by passiveness and undercontrol.[20]

External sources of stress (for example, the death of a spouse or loss of a job) are most likely beyond your control. To resolve stresses of this type, the best approach is to learn acceptance, coping, and self-management techniques. If your challenges are largely under your control, (problems such as poor parent-child relationships, spousal relationship, and financial difficulties), the best strategies would focus on learning mastery skills.

Put more simply, if a situation is within your control, you need to find new ways of dealing with it. If a situation is not within your control you need to learn acceptance and letting go.

Most people could benefit greatly from enhancing their skills in both mastery and acceptance, and every individual over the course of his or her adult life will require a continuous learning program that is personalized for his or her specific needs. Closely examining your results from the stress assessments in this chapter will suggest a curriculum of personal development that can make a very significant difference in your life and your future success.

Finding Solutions to Stress through Personal Growth

Personal growth—cognitive, behavioral, and spiritual—is a highly effective way to reduce stress arising from many different sources. Personal growth can be gained through classes, groups, and psychotherapy. A class in parenting skills, for example, can enhance order and harmony in your home and help you manage the demands of family life. Forgiving yourself and others who may contribute to your stress is an important part of stress reduction. You may find that once you have forgiven someone who has hurt you, you will need to learn to define clearer boundaries with that person or with other people in your life. This can involve learning new assertion skills.

5. Transform your thinking, your attitudes, and your interpretation of daily events to help you reduce your level of stress.

More than two thousand years ago, the Greek philosopher Heraclitus proclaimed that perception is a matter of choice. The way you respond to a situation, and the attitude you have toward it, directly affects the physiological impact of a stressful event. To reduce the negative effects on your mind and body, it is critical to understand that you have control over how you think and respond. Belief systems can create peace and harmony and reduce stress, or the opposite.

One principle you can choose to believe is that every upset contains a valuable learning experience that is central to your growth and maturity. You can also choose to believe that the person who created this upset has willingly sacrificed his own well-being to teach you this lesson.

For instance, it might be a parent or nemesis at work that is creating one upset after another for you. You can appreciate this person as someone willing to ruin his life, his relationships, and his happiness just to demonstrate to you how not to be. You can choose to see this person as teaching you this lesson: "Do not be angry, vindictive, resentful, and critical or you too will ruin your life like me."

"Health is inner peace" is a principle of attitudinal healing taught by Jerry Jampolsky, M.D., author of *Love Is Letting Go of Fear.* To achieve inner peace, it is necessary to let go of all resentments toward people in your life, including yourself. Forgiveness is a key to happiness. Letting go of resentments is a gradual process that can be emotionally difficult, as we receive many apparent but detrimental payoffs from holding resentments. An excuse for poor performance is one such payoff, and a sense of victimhood; a way of commiserating with others about why life does not work. "Perhaps they will change if I suffer enough," is the hope of this kind of martyr-dom. Although there are many payoffs to holding onto resentments, payoffs rob us of our well-being. Inner peace, health, and vitality await those who systematically resolve their resentments and critical judgments and find forgiveness as an ongoing way of being in the world.

Dr. Jampolsky teaches us to ask three questions when you feel upset.

1. What is upsetting me? Is it something in the present or is the situation reminding me of the past, or am I fearful of the future? This allows us to put the present into perspective.
2. Why am I holding onto the upset? Do I thrive on being a victim, or being helpless, or do I want to sacrifice my life and happiness in the hopes "they" will change?
3. What do I really want? I want peace, vitality, and creativity. I want to be a living example of these virtues to those I love.

Some people are naturally optimistic. They understand the value of giving a person or situation the benefit of the doubt and do not allow their minds to generate or dwell on negative thoughts. Others are conditioned at an early age to think the worst in any situation; this creates unnecessary stress. With these people, negative thinking occurs automatically, and they may not even be aware of their compulsion to view every situation in a negative light.

By learning to recognize patterns of thinking and feeling that create stress, and by understanding the impact of unhealthy attitudes, you can begin the process of transforming your thinking. Healthy attitudes can foster an inner peace that will help you attain success in other aspects of your life.

Creative Reinterpretation
Creative reinterpretation is another technique that works to vanquish a variety of stressors. By making the effort to

reinterpret a stressful event in a positive way, you can completely dissipate the stress of many everyday annoyances and frustrations.

Here is an example. Imagine you are on the freeway, driving home from a long day at the office, when another driver cuts you off. You could internalize the anger and frustration you feel, but this would trigger a chain reaction of stress-related damage to your body. Another choice would be to make up a story that creatively explains why this driver cut you off. For example, the driver's wife could be having a baby, and he is rushing to the hospital. A creative explanation will make his actions understandable; under the same circumstances, you would have done exactly as he did.

In truth, it is not possible to know why a random driver on the freeway behaves the way he does. The interpretation that there is a legitimate urgency behind the driver's actions is just as reasonable as the interpretation that the driver is rude. The best interpretation is one that will allow you to be calm in the situation.

Creative interpretation can be applied to any interpersonal situation. This technique is best used for situations that you want to learn to accept, rather than situations you want to learn to change and master. By combining this technique with assertion skills, you will be able to address your feelings calmly and solve problems in your relationships.

6. Adopt a consistent practice of meditation to reduce stress and build resilience to stress.

Meditation is one of the best ways to master stress before it masters you. Studies have demonstrated that people who meditate regularly have the highest level of success in preventing the harmful effects of stress.[21]

As is the case with all attitudinal techniques, to get positive results from meditation you must practice it on a consistent basis. Consistent practice helps prevent the accumulation of new stress by strengthening your mind, body, and spirit. Applying techniques such as meditation on a regular basis will give you the strength to manage your stress more effectively than an unconditioned individual.

Simple Breath Meditation Technique

Anyone can practice simple meditation techniques. You do not need special equipment, and you do not have to go to a special place to do it, although peace and quiet is conducive to the meditation process. One of the easiest forms of meditation is to count breaths. Sit quietly in a comfortable position, and close your eyes. Breathe in for a count of four, hold the breath in for a count of two, and then breathe out to a count of five. When you feel your mind wander, gently bring your attention back and focus on your breathing. After twenty minutes, you will be very relaxed, and you will find that your stress has dissipated.

The best and most intensive research on meditation has been done on Transcendental Meditation. This research shows that a person experiences an 18 percent to 20 percent decrease in oxygen consumption during the twenty minutes of meditation. Yet the brain receives over 20 percent more oxygen allowing for rejuvenation and revitalization of the brain. This means there is twice as much quality rest during meditation as during sleep, allowing you to efficiently dissolve built-up stress and fatigue. While meditating, the brain waves slow down and become coherent, indicating a distinct state of relaxed alertness.

This state of restfulness in the body and alertness in the mind is referred to as a fourth state of consciousness, since it is different from waking, sleeping, or dreaming states. Research suggests that this state of restful alertness may be as necessary for good health as sleeping or dreaming.[22] (See Appendix B for more information on meditation.)

7. Utilize the "love letter technique" to move quickly past stressful emotional states and restore acceptance and love to your relationships.

Following an argument or to relieve a recurring emotional upset with someone with whom you have a close personal or working relationship, you may find it useful to use the "love letter technique," popularized by John Gray, Ph.D., in his book *Men Are from Mars, Women Are from Venus.*

In this technique, you write the other person a letter that you do not deliver; the letter is a process for you. After an argument, it is common to become stuck in one of the negative emotions, such as anger, sadness, or fear. The purpose of writing the letter is to work through the range of emotions you may be feeling. The letter enables you to move past the anger, so that you can feel the sadness and grieve the loss. This in turn moves you into acceptance and love.

There are five levels of emotions to explore when writing a feeling letter. Begin each of the paragraphs with the following statements about your emotions:

- **Anger.** "I feel frustrated when . . . "
- **Sadness.** "I feel sad when . . . "
- **Fear.** "I feel afraid when . . . "
- **Remorse and apologies.** "I am sorry that . . . "
- **Love, understanding, gratitude, and forgiveness.** "I appreciate when . . . "

By moving through these emotions, you will dissolve the last barriers to love and acceptance. Finish your letter by completing this sentences: "Thank you for . . . " The love letter technique can help you feel better within a very short time and put situational stress behind you. Remember, it is not necessary to give the letter to the intended recipient. The primary purpose of this letter is to privately express and resolve your own feelings.

When you find it difficult to be loving, this is the perfect time to write a love letter. This technique will help you process your negative feelings and generate more positive loving feelings. This process should only take you twenty to thirty minutes. Don't focus on grammar, spelling, or punctuation. Let your feelings flow easily and naturally.

8. Achieve mastery over your time and routine to help you manage daily stress.

If you are not a highly organized person (and even if you are), time pressures can raise your stress level dramatically. When you are constantly feeling that there are not enough hours in the day to get things done, you may benefit from enrolling in a class to gain mastery in time management skills.

The following suggestions, adapted from the book *How to Get Control of Your Time and Your Life* by Alan Lakein, can help you change your approach toward time and get you started on the path to effective time management:

- Keep a daily "to do" list.
- Remember that probably only two out of ten things on the list are really worth doing.
- Focus on the important things; don't waste time on unimportant tasks, even if they are easy to complete.
- Reserve your most productive hours of the day for the tasks with the highest priority.
- Do the lowest priority tasks at those times when your energy level is the lowest.
- Keep to a firm routine to avoid indecision and wasted energy.
- Schedule time to relax, just as you would for an important appointment.

9. Experiment with mastery techniques and other stress reduction tools that may be a good fit for you.

If you have a job, a serious avocation or hobby, a family, or all three, you need to learn a diverse set of mastery skills to help you perform tasks efficiently and minimize the accumulation of stress.

For every life skill, there is a class or self-help book that can help you master it. Be honest with yourself in determining the areas in which you need assistance, and then get the help you need. One of the best things you can do to reduce stress is to improve yourself in the problem areas you have identified through the self-assessments you completed earlier in the chapter.

After carefully reviewing your assessment results, you may find that you could benefit from a class or book that teaches life skills in the following areas:

- Time management
- Parenting
- Financial planning
- Assertiveness training
- Vocational testing and training
- Leadership
- Public speaking
- Anger management
- Relationship skills
- Overcoming addictions

Find a Stress Coach

The more support you receive to adopt a new program, the better your chances for success. Surround yourself with people who encourage and support your stress reduction efforts. Create an accountability contract with a partner who is engaged in the same learning project or a supportive friend. Identify at least one person who will act as your coach. For this leadership position, choose someone who knows more about stress reduction than you do and can therefore provide wise guidance. Psychologists, teachers, spiritual leaders, and trained health coaches are all excellent choices for this role.

From Exercise to Creativity: Other Tools for Reducing Stress

The following stress reduction tools do not involve learning new cognitive or attitudinal skills, or changing your attitudes and beliefs to better accept your circumstances. These are body-oriented relaxation skills. Many physical techniques have demonstrated their effectiveness. Experiment with a variety of tools to learn what each can offer you. Your choice of stress reduction tools and techniques is a highly individualized one.

- **Exercise.** Exercise is a stress reduction tool that works for almost everyone. Yoga and tai chi are relaxing and meditative for people of all ages and any physical condition. Even people who are experiencing weak joints and severe muscle pain can achieve great results from water exercise, also known as hydrotherapy. For recommendations on how to get started with an exercise program and what to do, refer to the chapter on exercise.

- **Massage therapy.** Touch is highly therapeutic. Various forms of massage therapy are an effective stress reliever for many people. Not only does this ancient form of relaxation sedate the mind, it also provides a tremendous number of healing benefits for the body. During massage, a therapist applies pressure deep into the muscles and skin tissue. This process improves circulation, enhances cellular nutrition, and facilitates fresh oxygen flow to the brain, heart, and all the body tissues. Massage can lower blood pressure and heart rate during the therapy session.

- **Cranial electrotherapy stimulation.** Meditation works by altering your brain waves. If consistent practice of meditation is not easy for you, there is an effective tool called cranial electrotherapy stimulation (CES) that can help you produce positive brain wave changes without meditation. This treatment is simple and noninvasive. While undergoing CES treatment, you will feel a pleasant, relaxed feeling of well-being, which can last for hours or days after treatment. After one to two weeks of daily treatment, most patients notice an improvement in symptoms such as depression, insomnia, and anxiety. (See Appendix C for more information.)

- **Spa treatments.** Skin and body care treatments also involve touch. There is nothing like a day of personal pampering at a relaxing spa to neutralize your daily stress.

- **Creative pursuits.** Many people enjoy creative pursuits, such as music, painting, dancing, cooking, and writing, and find that these outlets take their minds away from their daily sources of stress.

- **Herbal therapy.** Adaptagens are herbs that balance the adrenal system and reduce the negative physical effects of stress.

- **Religious practices.** Prayer and religious rituals can also be a very constructive way to help manage stress and put your life's daily events into proper perspective. You may notice a dimension of stress in your life because a spiritual component is lacking. Spirituality involves a belief system or philosophy of life. It is important to think through and develop a theology or philosophy of life that will support positive attitudes in daily living.

  Spirituality and religion also create a connection to community. Research shows that people who attend regular religious services are healthier and live longer because they

feel connected to other people and find a sense of belong-
ing.[23] In a related statistic, research shows that happy
couples live longer than single people. The chapter entitled
Create Loving Romantic Relationships contains valuable
information on how you can improve your relationship
with your partner.

10. Document and execute a stress reduction plan.

Review the self-assessments you completed earlier to determine the sources of your stress and identify your stress
symptoms. This will tell you how your body is affected by
stress on a physiological and emotional level.

If you are experiencing frequent and severe headaches,
sleep disturbances, and gastrointestinal ailments, it may not
take much to convince you to implement a stress reduction
plan. Any scores of 4 or 5 in your completed assessments suggest an immediate need for reducing stress in those areas in
your life. Stress that appears in your attitudes and beliefs will
eventually create physical imbalance and disease.

It is important to manage your stress even when its effects
may be subtle; don't wait until you have substantial symptoms. In the beginning, pain, illness, and emotional distress
motivate us to reduce the stress in our lives. Later, the increasing joy of life and creativity motivate us. It is up to you to
motivate yourself.

To fully accept and adopt a stress reduction program, it is critical to document your personal plan. To make this process
easier, we have provided a template. Feel free to make multiple
copies of the form and use it to create your personal program.

When you have completed it, you will have developed a stress reduction plan ready for execution in the months to come.

Make Stress Reduction a Daily Activity

The human tendency, of course, is to implement self-improvement programs only after you are in a health crisis and then abandon them after you feel you have made some progress. Stress reduction should be an ongoing commitment, not a Band-Aid solution to fall back on when times get tough. It is necessary to make stress reduction as routine as brushing your teeth, eating, and showering each day. Once you make this transition, you will look forward to your routine and will find it easy to make it a priority in your daily activities. This is the best way to achieve success in managing your stress.

Update Your Plan Quarterly

Once per quarter, fill out a fresh copy of your stress reduction plan. Think carefully about any changes that have occurred in your life in the past three months. Have any new stressors been added, or have you gained newfound control over some sources of stress that were quite significant in the past?

Make a note of your three-month "anniversary" in your calendar. Committing to periodic updates of your plan will keep it fresh and interesting, motivate you, and greatly increase the likelihood that you will keep your stress under control for the long term.

PERSONAL STRESS REDUCTION PLAN

Date: _____

Your Name: _____

Your Life Crisis Unit (LCU) Score: _____

For every stress symptom you scored as 4 or 5, document them below for quick reference.

Primary Symptoms (Cognitive, emotional, behavorial, physiological, or social)	**Specific Symptoms** (Identified on the Assessment in Factor #1)	**Rating**
_____	_____	_____
_____	_____	_____
_____	_____	_____
_____	_____	_____
_____	_____	_____
_____	_____	_____
_____	_____	_____
_____	_____	_____
_____	_____	_____
_____	_____	_____
_____	_____	_____
_____	_____	_____
_____	_____	_____
_____	_____	_____
_____	_____	_____
_____	_____	_____
_____	_____	_____

For every source of stress you scored as 4 or 5, what specific actions will you take to reduce the stress?

Source of Stress	What Will You Do to Reduce the Stress?	When?
_____	_____	_____
_____	_____	_____
_____	_____	_____
_____	_____	_____
_____	_____	_____
_____	_____	_____
_____	_____	_____
_____	_____	_____
_____	_____	_____
_____	_____	_____
_____	_____	_____
_____	_____	_____
_____	_____	_____
_____	_____	_____

Who will you identify as your coach(es)? _____

_____

I will update this plan on (date): _____

Note: Make a copy of this form and update your plan every three months.

Chapter Summary

Chronic stress is a major factor in illness and disease. Unless it is resolved or managed, stress can lead to many debilitating and even life-threatening illnesses including cardiovascular disease, cancer, gastrointestinal and neurological disorders, anxiety, depression, and immune system imbalances.

Beliefs, attitudes, and emotions play an important role in stress. Simple negativity can confer a full range of stress-related symptoms; conversely, a positive attitude can give you some measure of immunity against the effects of stress. The first step to reducing stress in your life is to acknowledge those sources of stress that can be eliminated through a change in attitude or through acquiring new skills in living.

The ten recommendations described in this chapter can help you identify stress reduction strategies and techniques that may work best for you. The key is to select appropriate techniques and commit to a workable stress reduction plan.

Ten Practical Ways to Reduce Stress

1. Identify your current signs and symptoms of stress.
2. Identify external life events that may be causing you stress.
3. Identify your internal sources of stress.
4. Carefully examine the results of the stress assessment tests you have completed thus far to determine areas in which you could improve your skills of mastery and acceptance.
5. Transform your thinking, your attitudes, and your interpretation of daily events to help you reduce your level of stress.

6. Adopt a consistent practice of meditation to reduce stress and build resilience to stress.

7. Utilize the "love letter technique" to move quickly past stressful emotional states and restore acceptance and love to your relationships.

8. Achieve mastery over your time and routine to help you manage daily stress.

9. Experiment with mastery techniques and other stress reduction tools that may be a good fit for you.

10. Document and execute a stress reduction plan.

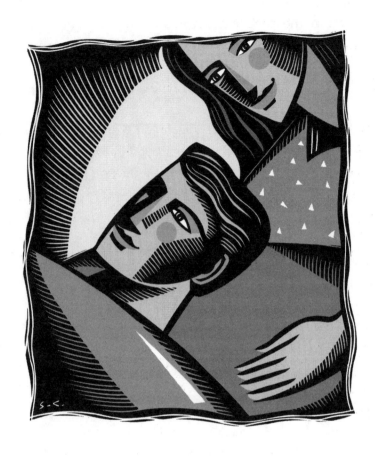

An unloving relationship accelerates the aging process; a loving relationship keeps the heart and soul young forever.

Key Factor Three

Create Loving Romantic Relationships
by Barbara Grossman, Ph.D. and Michael Grossman, M.D.

Barbara and I had a comfortable relationship during our first ten years of marriage. As we entered our thirties and our children were going to school, Barbara went back to graduate school to complete her Ph.D. and begin her professional life as an individual, marriage, and family therapist. As Barbara grew in independence, she also developed her own point of view, including new ideas and opinions about how our relationship should work. I found adjusting to this new development extremely difficult.

Getting beyond the power struggle of two strong and successful individuals who are trying to be in a romantic relationship can be very challenging. We've created some very practical ways for couples to get beyond their power struggle in order to create the quality of love that everyone wants in his or her life. This chapter is based on our real-life experiences and on the feedback received throughout twelve years of teaching relationship classes.

In twenty years of working with couples, Barbara finds that not every couple is ready to learn the skills necessary to develop a mature and satisfying marriage. Research shows that couples endure emotional hurt for an average of six years before seek-

ing relationship counseling. Even when one partner is ready to grow, the other may not be willing. One motivated partner can start the process and improve a relationship significantly. Ultimately, both partners need to collaborate to re-create their relationship. We suggest that you do not wait.

Couples and singles that take our classes are consistently enthusiastic about the resulting changes in their lives. The whole quality of your life changes when your primary relationship is filled with the sweetness of unlimited and unbounded love.

—Michael J. Grossman, M.D.

As a component of our personal wellness and vitality program, my husband Dave and I participated in a series of relationship classes facilitated by Drs. Michael and Barbara Grossman. We were enlightened and motivated by their presentation.

As with any significant behavioral change, this takes time and discipline. When we feel the need for a refresher, we reread this chapter. It has helped us stay focused on our most meaningful priorities in our life—our love, respect, and admiration for each other. It has elevated our relationship to new heights, and I'm confident it will do the same for yours.

—Jodi L. Jones

You may be thinking, why does a book about health contain a chapter on creating loving, romantic relationships? It is a medical fact that loving supportive relationships are essential for good health. Every major study on relationships and health agrees that divorced and separated people experience more physical and mental illness than those who are married.[1-4]

Married people live longer on average than those who are unmarried. Many studies show that divorced persons have twice the death rate of those married.[5-9] In addition, single or widowed men have two to six times the rate of death compared to married men.[10,11] Compared to single, married, and widowed individuals, the divorced group has the highest rates of acute and chronic illness.[12-14]

In addition, unhappily married people have poorer health than their single counterparts.[15,16] While no one knows for certain the reason that unmarried, divorced, and unhappily married people experience poorer health, the key factors, in our opinion, relate to the ongoing stress, hormonal changes,[17] and immune changes[18-20] that result from emotional upsets and social isolation. [21-25]

New research shows that even using negative language and an angry tone of voice when speaking with your partner can have a detrimental effect on your ability to ward off disease. Mental conflict has a deleterious effect on blood pressure, the heart, and the immune system.[26-29]

For example, in one five-year study, 10,000 men at high risk of developing angina were asked, "Does your wife show you her love?" Those who said "yes" had half the risk of experiencing angina.[30] Many large studies confirm that unhappily married men have much higher rates of heart disease than those who are happily married.[31,32]

By learning to communicate in a more loving, caring manner, you can improve both your relationship and your health.

Many people never learn how to make relationships fun, loving, joyful, and healthful. People manage all aspects of their lives—their careers, finances, families, and even leisure activities—but often do not take the time to sustain loving relationships.

Each of us is responsible for the quality of our relationships. To make yours a success, the most important thing to do is to place your relationship at the top of your list of priorities in your life. Both partners have to pay close attention to the relationship, devote time to it on a daily basis, and do whatever it takes to ensure that they are able to spend adequate amounts of quality time together. Taking responsibility for your relationship may sound like a very demanding process, but when your relationship is satisfying on an emotional, physical, and spiritual level, it will increasingly become a source of joy and fun and vibrant health for both of you.

During courtship, creating pleasurable experiences is almost second nature, and both partners find it easy to devote the time and effort necessary to deepen the relationship. Later, when you make the transition into something more permanent, the pressures and responsibilities of life can overwhelm you, and you can forget what brought you together in the first place. The secret is to continue courting behavior, even when you are surrounded by the distractions of everyday life, not to mention crying babies and dirty diapers. Taking out time for romantic dates and creating opportunities for intimate sharing is vital to maintaining a healthy romantic connection.

John Gottman, one of the most esteemed researchers in the field of marriage success and failure, describes four behaviors that destroy a marriage: critical anger, contempt, fearful defensiveness, and emotional withdrawal. These four behaviors represent the two extremes that can occur in a troubled relationship: On one hand is contempt and anger, and on the other is indifference and emotional distance.[33]

In teaching relationship classes for over twelve years, we have found that appreciating the differences between men and women is crucial to creating intimate, caring romantic relationships.

The Differences between Men and Women

Medical researchers find clear differences between the human male and female brains. The male brain has fewer connections between the right and left hemispheres, while the female brain has rich connections. In general, the right hemisphere controls the left side of the body and relates to our artistic, intuitive, emotional qualities. The left hemisphere controls the right side of the body and generally relates to logic, language, and mathematics. Men are basically more specialized in focusing on the dominant left hemisphere of logic and linear goal-oriented thought. Women are more capable, in general, of moving between the two hemispheres in doing things that involve both emotion and thinking.[34]

This can be understood in terms of the evolution of the roles of men and women. For millions of years, men were the hunters. Tracking and killing a large animal involves the utmost concentration and focus on one goal and one task while suppressing emotional distractions. Women, on the other hand, simultaneously gathered food, laughed, played, supervised the children, prepared meals, and watched for predators.[35]

This anthropological history explains why women are typically more adept at moving back and forth between feeling and thinking. Women are generally less linear in how they create relationships. When we look at a group of women having lunch together, their conversation moves from feeling to thinking in an easy, flowing process with very little problem solving. In listening to a group of men having lunch together, we will typically hear a discussion that is linear and problem oriented, usually not about feelings.

We agree with relationship expert Gary Smalley, Ph.D., author of several relationship books, that women have a tendency to say almost twice as many words per day as men. These behaviors may be structured in the differences between the male and female brains.

It is neither good nor bad that men and women are different in this way. However, understanding and accepting these differences is crucial to creating loving romantic relationships. In the most personal part of the relationship, a woman needs to be able to safely express her feminine self and a man needs to be able to express himself without her criticism or judgment. In other aspects of the relationship, you can problem solve and partner in an egalitarian mode. However, the sharing of feelings is very delicate. We need to share our commonalties as well as our differences.

We can create processes in our relationships that allow a man and woman to safely share together, understand their differences, and express desires for new behaviors that are perceived as loving and caring.

Relationship Skills for Women: Making Requests

Men and women have different needs in a relationship. In twelve years of teaching relationship classes, we have found most women would like more attention and emotional intimacy from their men. Unfortunately, these kinds of desires are characteristically vague. To get their needs met, women must learn to ask for what they want in very specific terms. This usually means expressing specific pleasurable desires.

Many women find it very difficult to request specific pleasurable behaviors from their partners. Since men are not adept at reading a woman's wishes from vague or unspoken cues, they need to be told what they can do to make their partner happy, and then need to feel that any efforts they have put forth have been genuinely appreciated. Having their efforts acknowledged and appreciated helps to satisfy the need that a man has to feel respected and admired for his ability to produce and deliver for his woman.

When a woman acquires the skill of making behavioral requests and appreciating her man's response, she can receive the attention she craves, and the man can receive the respect and admiration he seeks. Mastery of these skills can make the relationship work at an optimal level for both partners.

Relationship Skills for Men: Sharing Feelings

Men often have less trouble asking for what they want, but they usually need to learn to share feelings. To maximize the success of their relationship, couples must share feelings. In turn, successful sharing is dependent on creating a safe, comfortable environment in which both partners can be open in expressing deep feelings.

Sharing from the heart should be at the center of your life together. You need to create time for it, and share what is important to you in a calm, respectful way.

The way in which each gender approaches the sharing process reflects the essential differences between women and men. Women need to learn to share their feelings in a calm, rational way instead of dramatizing them. Men need to learn to share their feelings without giving in to the temptation to offer unwanted advice. Men also need to say, "Ouch, that hurts" when something emotionally uncomfortable occurs.

As stated earlier, the key to creating loving romantic relationships is your commitment to making your relationship one of the most important values in your life. Make the relationship more important than a fleeting urge to express your anger or your desire to win an argument at the expense of your partner. It is important to note that one of the primary factors involved in relationship demise is control, the need to exert control over your partner's thoughts, opinions, and actions.

The ten recommendations in this chapter will help you make dramatic improvements in your relationship skills. By putting into practice the ten recommendations for relationships that follow, you will be able to prevent relationship stress from damaging your health and profoundly diminishing your joy in living.

Although we focus on creating loving, romantic relationships in this chapter, it is just as important to recognize the value of developing loving relationships with your family members and respectful and caring relationships with your friends and close co-workers. Strained, disrespectful, and abusive relationships of any type can create stress. However, strategies for developing healthy relationships beyond romantic relationships are quite different and are not the purpose of this chapter.

The following assessment will score your skill in creating a loving romantic relationship.

Mastery of Relationship Assessment

For each question that follows, write your response with a number that corresponds to the key below. Add up the total score at the end and assess your skill in creating loving romantic relationships.

Scoring Key
1 = agree strongly or always true
2 = agree or generally true
3 = not sure
4 = disagree or generally not true
5 = disagree strongly or never

For men and women:

_____ I make time with my partner to discuss sensitive topics several times each week.

_____ I do not spring surprise attacks on my partner. Whenever I have a grievance with my partner, I ask for the best time to sit down and discuss it.

_____ I rarely express raw, unprocessed anger to my partner.

_____ I avoid using an angry tone when speaking to my partner.

_____ I am aware that anger is based on old emotional hurts.

_____ I am gentle about my partner's insecurities.

_____ I reserve at least one day a week for a personal night out with my partner.

_____ I share feeling, hopes, disappointments, and expectations with my partner during intimate sharing time at least twice a week.

For men:

_____ I always ask my partner if she wants me just to listen or to give advice.

_____ I am attuned to the subtle signs and desires of my partner.

_____ I listen carefully to what makes her happy.

_____ I do many little things to show my partner I love her.

_____ I never criticize or belittle my partner's requests for things that make her happy.

_____ I am careful to clarify the details of my partner's desires for things that make her happy.

For women:

_____ I am enthusiastic with my thanks for anything my partner does to try and please me.

_____ I ask for specific pleasurable behaviors for my man to do for me.

_____ I thank my partner enthusiastically for the things he does to make my requests happen.

_____ I never demand or threaten when I make requests for things that make me happy.

_____ I do not stand over my partner and watch closely to see if he is fulfilling my requests properly.

_____ I never get irritable or angry about waiting for my requests to be fulfilled.

Now add your scores for each question to assess your skill in creating loving romantic relationships.

RELATIONSHIP SCORE RESULTS

14 to 20   You have a great mastery in relationships.

21 to 34   You have good relationship skills but need some fine-tuning.

31 to 42   Your relationship can be more pleasurable—skills need improving.

43 to 50   You can do much better and have more joy in your relationship by using these recommendations.

51 or more   It is essential to practice the ten practical ways to change your relationship to create joy and pleasure.

The following recommendations have been categorized by (1) for men, (2) for both women and men and (3) for women, and By following these ten practical methods, you will be on your way to creating a loving romantic relationship with your spouse or significant other.

Ten Practical Ways for Creating Loving Romantic Relationships

1. (For men) Do many little things that show you love your partner and demonstrate your attention to her feminine qualities.

From a woman's point of view, buying her a new car and giving her a red rose weigh equally in her perceptions that you love her. Many men make the mistake of thinking that one colossal extravagance will cover them for a multitude of sins or months of indifference. In his woman's eyes, the man who brings home a rose a week and caresses and hugs daily is miles ahead of the man who splurges on big expensive gifts only at birthdays and holidays.

2. (For men) Listen carefully when your partner appears to be making some sort of request and make sure to draw her out for specifics about precisely what is going to make her happy.

Imagine a woman who tells her partner that she would like more attention. This vague request could encompass anything from "Please stop reading the newspaper at the dinner table" to "Let's go out dancing one day next week." Probe for specifics. Take the time to discover what she really wants every time her request seems vague.

Men must avoid belittling a woman's request or making it sound unimportant. When it comes to choosing an activity, men generally like to build or create things and be practical. Generally, we encourage women to express requests that are less practical, more spontaneous, and more focused on enjoying the moment.

You have to expect that your woman's requests will not fit into a manly worldview; she may want to do something that, from your perspective, seems completely nonproductive. She may ask you to stroll through the park with her, or go out and look at the stars. She may want you to kiss and hug her before leaving every morning and after coming home every evening. Her wants may seem silly or nonsensical to you, but do yourself and your relationship a favor and honor her requests. Make your partner's desires important; ignoring them will injure the flow of love in your relationship.

3. (For women and men) Do not spring surprise attacks. Make appointments to discuss sensitive topics or things that have been bothering you.

It is common for one partner to spring a hot-button conversation on the other at an inconvenient or high-stress time. An example of a "surprise attack" is when a woman begins to verbally attack her partner on his arrival home from a difficult day at work. If he has lost a major account and been reprimanded by his boss, this is precisely the wrong time for the woman to air her grievances. An impromptu discussion at this time will very likely cause tempers to flare and create resentment on both sides.

Contrast this with a conversation in which the partner with a complaint or request arranges an appointment in advance; both parties are receptive to the idea of working together toward a solution. There are no surprises, and setting the appointment results in a completely different, and infinitely more positive, experience.

Many men make the mistake of offering unsolicited advice to a woman, seeking to provide a quick fix to a problem when she is only trying to get something off her chest. When the woman requests an appointment, the man should ask first if she wants him to listen only or to offer advice. Proffering unwanted advice makes a woman feel controlled, unheard, and not cherished.

4. (For women and men) Make time for nonjudgmental, ten-minute sharing sessions several times a week.

You would be surprised how much ground you can cover and how deep you can go in only ten minutes, when that time is devoted exclusively to discussing intimate feelings and critical issues. If you pursue these brief sharing sessions consistently, you may find that you have learned more about how your partner thinks and feels within a few months than you have managed to discover during decades of marriage.

When the two of you are sharing, listen but do not judge. Let your partner have the floor without interruption for five minutes; then you can take your turn. Focusing attention and not reacting during a sharing session creates that safe environment you and your partner need to feel comfortable and open in expressing deep feelings. If you interrupt and act defensively when your partner shares, or you discount every point or make your partner feel stupid for bringing an issue up, communication between the two of you will be stifled.

Why limit sharing sessions to only ten minutes? Women are able to share their intimate feelings for extended periods of time; generally speaking, most women have developed their sharing skills. For most men, intimate sharing will be a whole new ball game.

Men need short sessions in order to feel comfortable sharing. If a session ends abruptly with business left unfinished, do not insist on finishing what was started. Instead, schedule an appointment for another sharing session in the near future. Women, if you are patient with this process, you will gradually stretch the depth and consistency of emotional intimacy in your relationship.

5. (For women and men) Commit to managing, rather than expressing, your anger.

In all relationships, anger must be managed. It is helpful and constructive to express a feeling such as sadness, but expressing your raw, unprocessed anger is usually destructive.

Anger never stands on its own. There is always some other emotion behind it. As Jerry Jampolsky, M.D., so eloquently states in his book *Love Is Letting Go of Fear*, "You are never upset for the reason you think."[36] Upsets are always related to past experiences. The present situation reactivates old hurts, fears, sadness, and losses. If we can share prior experiences, typically those from many years ago and even from childhood, we can begin to understand the sensitivities in the present situation and start to unravel the emotional tangles we are presently experiencing.

To ensure healthy, positive communication, reach beneath the anger and express the sadness, sense of loss, or fears that underlie it. Before reflexively sharing your anger in a hostile way, it is helpful to discover what your anger is trying to teach you. Share how old you feel during an emotional encounter. For example, if your spouse is criticizing you, explain how you feel like you are ten years old again and your mother is yelling at you for not doing something her way. Sharing feelings in this manner will strengthen your bond. The alternative is venting your anger and eroding trust. This may eventually destroy the relationship.

6. (For women and men) Acknowledge and be gentle about your partner's insecurities.

Gender notwithstanding, we all have our sensitive spots, areas of insecurity and self-doubt that are very tender. For example, men are often sensitive to criticism about their ability to do things, fix things, achieve things, and fulfill a woman's desires. Many women are insecure about their attractiveness—their body shape, hair, complexion, and weight.

Men, if you want your relationship to flourish, do not give your partner reasons to doubt your willingness to do things to please her. Notice and appreciate her, pay attention to everything she says, and be generous with your affection. When she takes the time to get dressed up, make a special point of telling her just how great she looks. Be genuine and say it because you mean it.

And women, be sure to respect and appreciate the effort your man is willing to make for you, however small it may be. Know that he is willing and wanting to please you. Do not disregard his attempts. This will only discourage him from trying to please you in the future.

7. (For women) Appreciate any progress your partner makes in the direction of fulfilling your request, even if it is only a fraction of what you wanted or expected.

Making requests is an art, not a science. The act of making and fulfilling requests strengthens the romantic relationship, honoring the feminine qualities of the woman and the masculine qualities of the man. A request that is feminine in nature may be best suited to enhance the romantic relationship; for example, requesting a romantic dinner or a walk on the beach, versus asking the man to take out the garbage. Be aware, that the request needs to be for something that will make you happy; its purpose is to foster the romantic relationship.

A request is not a demand. The man has a choice of whether to fulfill the request or not, and your partner may want to respectfully negotiate the terms of your request. Do not judge your partner harshly if he wishes to deliver some variation of your request, according to a timetable that is more convenient for him.

For the woman, a request is an opportunity to persuade, by attraction. Early on in a relationship, women know how to magnetize and compel a man to get what they want; this is what lends excitement to the courtship phase. When the relationship becomes more permanent, however, women seem to forget how to attract and influence their partner. This takes the magic and mystery out of the relationship and makes things a lot more dull and boring than they need to be.

Be effusive in your appreciation and gratitude for whatever your partner does for you in fulfilling a request. Never criticize or correct him if he delivers a result that you consider incomplete or somehow lacking. Give him your sincere thanks at the time he completes any action to fulfill your desire, and make a new request at a later time. This will give him the opportunity to generate a result that is more in line with your expectations.

8. (For women) Ask nicely for what you want. Start with simple requests to train your relationship gradually.

Ask nicely whenever you make a request. Emphasize to your man how much you will appreciate it when he has fulfilled your request. These are the keys to making him want to do things for you.

No matter what he does or says in response to your request, do not react to it. He may grunt, he may complain, he may turn up the volume on the football game, and he may even offer excuses. But these sometimes irritating noises and sound effects only indicate that he is revving up his engine, getting ready to perform for you. The worst thing you could do is respond with anger, which to him sounds like you are complaining before he has even had a chance to get started.

An important corollary to this is to start out small and slow. Motivate your partner to produce good results for you by starting him off with easy tasks. He will be much more receptive to a task that he can complete in an hour or less than to a complex request that could take months of effort or requires a large financial commitment. If your request is a large and complex one, try breaking it down into smaller tasks and presenting them one at a time.

9. (For women) Be patient and enthusiastic while waiting for your partner to fulfill your request— do not micromanage your partner.

Although it may be against your natural instincts, it is important to be patient and enthusiastic once you make a request of your partner. This means not demanding that your request be completed within your time frame and to your "specifications." Provide him with advance notice and allow him to organize the request into his schedule.

Do not doubt your partner's ability to deliver what you want. If he says he will fix the leaky faucet for you, and water starts to flood out from the sink, resist all temptation to call a plumber yourself or point out his lack of skills as a handyman. Always encourage him in his efforts to be your "knight in shining armor." The male ego is far more fragile than it appears to be.

Also, it is important not to micromanage your partner as he acts on your request. If you are feeling any frustration regarding his performance, find a way to manage yourself so that you do not express it. Do not criticize him if he does not do the job exactly as you would like to see it done. Do not get angry with him as time passes without him finishing the task, or even starting it. The best and most productive stance for you to take, the position most likely to lead you to getting what you want, is one of telling him of your eager anticipation.

Of course, if he has not begun to act on your request in a reasonable amount of time, arrange an appointment to discuss the situation (see #3).

10. **(For women and men) Communicate your own point of view calmly and honestly and make a sincere effort to draw out and understand your partner's point of view.**

Good relationships are built on good communication. If you want to be heard and understood, you need to express yourself calmly and leave your anger out of it. Always initiate sensitive or emotionally charged discussions by making the other person feel that you have some understanding of his or her point of view. A good opener might be, "I know you've been upset with me about the way I handled _____ (the situation)." Communicating an awareness of the other's feelings up front supports a safe conversation and will allow your partner to hear your point of view without getting defensive or angry.

Romantic love has the potential of opening our hearts to a quality of love that is truly divine. It does require that we give up the blocks and restrictions in our beliefs and attitudes that hold us back from deeply loving our partner.

Chapter Summary

Men and women are different when it comes to relationships. The most critical skill for a woman to develop in order to improve the relationship is to learn to request specific things that her man can do to make her happy, and then express pleasure in receiving what he gives her. The most important relationship skill a man needs to learn is to be sensitive about feelings. When both partners make the effort to master these core skills, their reward will be a relationship abundant in joy and fun.

Remember to rescore yourself at monthly intervals. When you think you are doing well, ask your partner to score you and discuss the results together. Continue to rescore yourself and discuss the results with your partner every three months until you reach mastery in romantic relationships.

The ten recommendations described in this chapter can help improve your relationship skills dramatically and prevent relationship stress from eroding your health. Practice them and be patient with each other. Gradually all of us can individuate, develop, and mature into people who bring great joy to each other.

Ten Practical Ways to Create Loving Romantic Relationships

1. (For men) Do many little things that show you love your partner and demonstrate your attention to her feminine qualities.

2. (For men) Listen carefully when your partner appears to be making some sort of request, and make sure to draw her out for specifics about precisely what is going to make her happy.

3. (For men and women) Do not spring surprise attacks. Make appointments to discuss sensitive topics or things that have been bothering you.

4. (For men and women) Make time for nonjudgmental ten-minute sharing sessions several times a week.

5. (For men and women) Commit to managing, rather than expressing, your anger.

6. (For men and women) Acknowledge and be gentle about your partner's insecurities.

7. (For women) Appreciate any progress your partner makes in the direction of fulfilling your request, even if it is only a fraction of what you wanted or expected.

8. (For women) Ask nicely for what you want. Start with simple requests to train your relationship gradually.

9. (For women) Be patient and enthusiastic while waiting for your partner to fulfill your request—do not micromanage your partner.

10. (For men and women) Communicate your own point of view calmly and honestly and make a sincere effort to draw out and understand your partner's point of view.

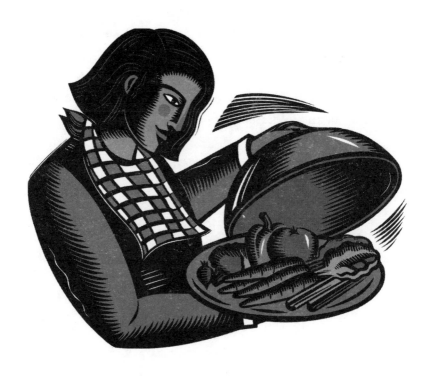

Healthy eating requires discipline and planning—the rewards will be worth the investment.

Key Factor Four
Eat Balanced, Nutritious Meals

When I was growing up in a small town in Michigan, I ate a typical all-American Midwestern diet consisting of what many consider comfort foods: steaks, baked potatoes with sour cream and butter, pizza with extra cheese, pepperoni, and an extra thick crust, hamburgers, chili dogs, potato chips, and many other damaging foods. When prepackaged meals entered the grocery stores, I indulged in a variety of processed foods. Does this diet sound familiar?

I was not embarrassed to be called "junk-food Jodi"; thanks to my high metabolism, I looked completely healthy and fit my entire life. What I didn't know was that eating all those foods contributed to my autoimmune diseases. Despite my outside appearance, my body was slowly attacking itself and thoroughly confusing my immune system.

As a living testimonial, I am thrilled to share these practical ways to optimize your nutrition. After reading this chapter, you will have the knowledge to make informed decisions about your dietary choices, giving you the opportunity to optimize, not jeopardize, your health by eating balanced nutritious meals.

Bon appétit.

—*Jodi L. Jones*

At New York University Medical School in the early 1970s, the study of nutrition consisted of a single lecture on protein, fat, carbohydrates, and a few essential vitamins and minerals. Since then, there has been an explosion of knowledge about new categories of nutrients, such as carotenoids, flavanoids, lycopene, lutein, proanthocyanadins, and a multiplicity of other phytonutrients. Today, there is also new knowledge about anti-inflammatory and proinflammatory diets.

The nutritional conferences I regularly attend to keep up with these breakthroughs are populated by naturopathic doctors, chiropractors, acupuncturists, nutritionists, and a few medical doctors. Nutritional approaches to health are too low tech and time consuming for many medical doctors. Nevertheless, it is the foundation of good health.

Taking supplements prescribed by your health practitioner can be very important to your health, but this does not replace healthy eating. There are still many undiscovered nutrients in fresh whole foods.

Nutrition can be a confusing topic to study. This chapter will present clear and practical information to help you create your vitality program.

—Michael J. Grossman, M.D.

The relationship between diet and disease has been scientifically studied for centuries. The concept of proper nutrition resulting in better health is certainly not a breakthrough idea. In fact, in 390 A.D. Hippocrates stated, "Let food be your medicine and medicine be your food."

The purpose of this chapter is to provide a foundation for a healthful diet based on nutritious foods. It is not designed as an absolute prescription to cure all ailments. Nor does it describe the optimum diet for those wanting to lose excessive weight. There is no absolute "right" diet. There are many diets and weight loss programs that focus on reducing caloric intake, eliminating fat, and avoiding carbohydrates. Some recommend an optimal diet based on your blood type; others have been devised based on your body shape.

There are many fad diets being promoted, many of which hold merit and effectiveness for some period of time, not necessarily forever. There are many destructive diets we label as "yo-yo diets" where you lose fat weight with muscle, then gain more fat weight, and once again lose more weight, muscle, and fat; overall more muscle is lost. A natural result of a healthful balanced diet, as detailed throughout this chapter, should be gradual and sustained weight loss or weight gain if that is what your body needs, while maintaining muscle mass. The nutrition recommendations described herein are foundational and appropriate to maintain long-term, consistent good health and well-being.

The chapters on supplementation and a healthy kitchen are closely related in content, so for best results read and refer to all three of these chapters. By doing so, you will understand what to eat, how best to prepare it, and the critical need to supplement what you eat with quality vitamins and minerals.

Balancing Macronutrients: Protein, Carbohydrate, and Fat

The first step to success in optimizing nutrition is to be aware of everything you are putting into your body to ensure that every meal is both nutritious and contains balanced amounts of macronutrients (food sources needed by your body in large amounts): protein, carbohydrate, and (healthy) fat. The amount of each macronutrient depends on your current health condition and objectives. The following provides a general range, based on percent of total calories, according to your health goals:

	Fat Burning	Muscle Building	Weight Maintenance
Protein:[1]	30%	40%	20%
Carbohydrates:[2]	40%	30%	50–60%
Fats:	30%	30%	20–30%

Food Allergies or Intolerances

Throughout this chapter, we will recommend various types of foods. It is important to realize that not everyone can tolerate or benefit equally from the same types of foods. Some people are allergic to fish, others to seeds and nuts, and many have reactions to various fruits and vegetables, as well as wheat and dairy.

Food allergies are common and present a myriad of symptoms. They are often misdiagnosed. Whether you self-diagnose your food allergies or seek the help of a nutrition-focused health practitioner, it is important to make this a priority in your overall quest for optimum health and vitality. For guidance, please read the chapters on detoxification and fatigue. The

---

1. If you have kidney or liver problems, consume less than 20 percent of your calories from animal protein, as this form of protein taxes these organs.
2. Consumption of complex carbohydrates or low-glycemic carbohydrates, not simple carbohydrates such as potatoes, white rice, white flour, pasta, and refined sugar.

recommendations offered in these two chapters will provide a good basis to begin self-diagnosing your food allergies.

Relevant Concepts

The topic of nutrition is extensive and complex. Hundreds of books have been written addressing the many factors associated with proper diet and nutrition. For the purpose of this chapter, it is helpful to have a basic understanding of the following concepts and their role in nutrition.

- **Caloric intake.** The amount of calories an individual should consume daily varies based on gender, age, activity level, and current weight. The average, moderately active woman between twenty-five and fifty years of age should consider 1,600 to 2,000 calories per day. The average, moderately active man between twenty-five to fifty years of age should consider 2,200 to 2,600 calories per day. If your goal is to lose weight, caloric intake should be reduced. Before beginning a weight-loss program, be sure to consult with an experienced licensed health practitioner.

- **Portion control.** When consuming your meals, be mindful of the portion of a given food you are serving or consuming. Americans are famous for "super sizing" their food portions. One of the simplest steps to reduce the quantity of your food intake is to use a smaller plate or bowl than you would normally use.

- **Hormones.** Hormones are powerful in determining whether you burn fat or store fat. Insulin can be viewed as your body's fat-storage hormone. The pancreas secretes insulin in response to elevated blood sugar (glucose) levels, primarily from ingesting excessive carbohydrates in a meal. One of its main functions is to decrease blood glucose levels when they get too high. Glucagon is completely opposite from insulin and is considered a fat-burning hormone. Glucagon is also released by the pancreas, primarily in response to diminished blood sugar. It is also released in response to eating protein. By utilizing stored body fat for energy, glucagon helps maintain stable blood sugar levels.

■ **Glycemic index.** It is important to control glucose levels in order to reduce excess insulin production. The glycemic index is a system that rates how quickly certain foods increase blood sugar levels and how quickly the body responds by bringing levels back to normal. The higher the number, the faster the food raises blood sugar, resulting in insulin surges. This aggravates diabetes and hypoglycemia. (Refer to Appendix D for the Glycemic Index table.)

■ **Antinutrients.** There are many foods consumed that actually rob your body of essential nutrients. Additionally, many environmental toxins and lifestyle choices are considered antinutrients. The following are some of the antinutrients you should try to avoid for optimum nutrition:

• Pollution
• Foods grown with pesticides
• Processed foods
• Fried foods
• Caffeine
• Alcohol
• Tobacco
• Sugar
• Most polyunsaturated fats

The ten recommendations that follow will provide you with a foundation for a healthful diet based on nutrient-rich foods. Remember, food is medicine. Consume it wisely and mindfully and heal yourself. It is possible to literally eat your way to maximized health and vitality.

Ten Practical Ways to Eat Balanced, Nutritious Meals

1. Optimize your protein intake. Virtually eliminate red meat and animal fat from your diet; instead consume fish, poultry, and plant sources of protein (soy beans, legumes, nuts, and grains).

Protein is required by your body to build muscle and connective tissue and is critical for brain development. The twenty-five amino acids—different building blocks of protein—are critical for cell renewal and are used to make hormones, enzymes, antibodies, and neurotransmitters that help transport substances around the body.

A discussion about protein must include a brief mention of fat, since many sources of animal protein contain high levels of "bad" fats, as well as harmful hormones and pesticides. As has been highly publicized in the media, animal meat (especially beef) and dairy products (milk, eggs, cheese, and butter) contain high levels of saturated fats that cause hardening of the arteries and increase other health risks. In addition to fat, cows, pigs, and sheep have a high exposure to hormones, antibiotics, and pesticides. These animals ingest pesticides that are used in growing their feed and receive doses of hormones to increase growth rates and maximize milk yields. Antibiotics are used in exorbitant amounts to treat the plethora of diseases contracted by these animals as well.

That being said, the news on red meat is not all bad. Red meat contains CLA (conjugated linoleic acid), which has been shown to be helpful in fighting cancer as well as losing weight. Most of the red meat available today is from grain-fed livestock kept in pens; a better choice would be meat from free-range herds eating grass. Grass-fed herds produce more nutritious meat than grain-fed stock. When you have a craving for red meat, select the highest grade, organic when possible, and opt for the leanest cut.

Dairy products, a popular source of protein, also contain hormones and pesticides. Many people are allergic to dairy products (lactose intolerant) and have difficulty digesting milk sugar, resulting in unnecessary flatulence, bloating, and belching. Other allergy symptoms include constipation, irritability, fatigue, diarrhea, and respiratory problems.[1,2]

Cow's milk has been linked to many forms of cancer, including breast, prostate, and colon cancer. Milk has also been associated with heart disease and diabetes.[3] Cutting back on dairy can reduce saturated fat in your diet and minimize many serious health risks. Instead of dairy, it is better for most people to consume soy products that provide a healthy form of protein. Although nonfat milk and yogurt may be acceptable in moderate amounts, try substituting soymilk and soy yogurt.

Soy has been found to help mitigate many perimenopausal and menopausal symptoms[4,5] and has been shown to lower cholesterol;[6,7] compounds in soy called isoflavones may offer significant protection against common forms of cancer.[8–10]

Free-range organic chicken and turkey are good substitutes for red meat, as they are subjected to lesser amounts of hormones, antibiotics, and pesticides. Additionally, skinless chicken breasts and turkey contain virtually no saturated fat. How you prepare and cook your poultry determines how healthy it will be for you. Do not deep-fry or use a charcoal barbeque grill, as these methods are toxic. Instead, for the healthiest cooking results, you should steam, lightly sauté in extra-virgin olive oil, or bake/roast your skinless chicken breasts and turkey.

Egg whites are a good source of protein; it is the yolk that contains most of the cholesterol. However, the yolk also contains the "good fat," B vitamins, and other important nutrients. If your cholesterol levels are within a safe range, it is beneficial to eat the entire egg periodically, provided it is prepared in a healthful way, poached or sunny side up, not scrambled. To get the most nutritious eggs, look for those from chickens that are fed a diet of fish; these eggs are fortified with healthy omega-3 fat. Eggs from free-range organic farms are also healthier, with higher quality nutrients and fewer pesticides and hormones.

Fish is also a healthy source of protein and, depending on the fish, a good source of healthy omega-3 fats. However, to avoid the harmful toxic effects of mercury found in most large fish that swim in mercury-laden polluted ocean waters, it is best to choose smaller fish that are lower in the food chain, such as herring, mackerel, sardines, or fresh farm-raised salmon. The mercury problem is amplified in the case of large fish, such as swordfish, shark, and tuna, which eat other smaller fish, therefore resulting in compounded mercury consumption. To prevent absorption of mercury, take at least 50 mcg of selenium while you are eating these larger fish.

Fish that are farm raised should not contain mercury, since what these fish eat can be better controlled. Farm-raised fish are lower in omega-3 oils, however. Additional healthy sources of protein include those from plant sources: legumes (peas, beans, and lentils), nuts, grains, some vegetables (spinach, corn, broccoli, and potatoes), and soybeans.

The amount of protein in each type of food described above varies greatly. Typically men and weight lifters need more protein in their diets than women and those who don't lift weights.

2. Optimize your carbohydrate intake. Eat fresh organic fruits and vegetables, as well as whole grains and beans.

Carbohydrates provide the main fuel for the body. They come in two forms: "fast releasing," such as those in sugar, honey, malts, sweets, and most refined and processed foods, and "slow releasing," such as in whole grains, fresh fruits, beans, and vegetables. The latter foods contain more complex carbohydrate and/or more fiber, both of which help to slow down the release of sugar. Fast-releasing carbohydrates tend to give a sudden burst of energy followed by a slump, while slow-releasing carbohydrates provide more sustained energy and are therefore more beneficial. The frequent consumption of fast-releasing carbohydrates contributes to serious health conditions such as attention deficit disorder, diabetes, hypoglycemia, and digestive problems.

When choosing fruits and vegetables as your carbohydrate source, it is best to buy organic produce—it is grown with virtually no toxic fertilizers and pesticides. Commercial fertilizers leach valuable vitamins and trace minerals out of the soil, resulting in nutrient-deficient produce.

Follow this hierarchy when considering which form of fruits and vegetables to buy:

- Best for you: **Fresh organic**

  Fresh organic fruits and vegetables are best eaten within a few days of purchase to attain maximum nutritional benefit. Remember the saying: Good food goes bad; bad food lasts forever. This adage applies not only to fruits and vegetables, but to basically all foods. The better it is for you, typically, the faster the food will spoil. The worse it is for you, the longer "shelf life" it has due to preservatives, chemicals, canning processes, and so on. It is best to consume at least five servings of fresh fruits and vegetables every day.

- Second best: **Dried**

  Rotate your consumption of fresh fruit with dried fruit. Although the fiber from dried fruit is a good remedy for constipation, the process of drying fruit produces a higher concentration of natural sugar, as much as six times more. The extra sugar is easy to assimilate and provides an excellent source of energy; however, those wanting to lose weight, or who are diabetic or hypoglycemic, should especially avoid dried fruit. Also, dried fruits have less vitamin C per gram than fresh fruits, except for dried pears which have twice as much vitamin C in dried pears as ripe, raw pears. Dried plums (prunes) are rich in vitamin A, potassium, and magnesium. Dried apricots are high in vitamin A, iron, magnesium, and potassium.

- Third best: **Frozen**

  The process of freezing fruits and vegetables varies greatly and impacts their nutritional value. Fruits that are frozen immediately after being picked offer the highest nutritional benefit. The same applies to vegetables; the best method is to quickly blanch the vegetables (to blanch, first boil in filtered water for a minute or two, then immediately immerse in ice water and drain). Store-bought frozen fruits and vegetables are less nutrient rich. Additionally, prolonged storage in the freezer reduces nutrient levels.

- Last option: **Canned**

  Canning generally involves some heating during processing, which destroys a large portion of the nutrients. The exception to this rule occurs with tomatoes, which are just as nutritious canned as fresh. Both forms contain the antioxidant lycopene, a cancer-fighting agent.

How should you prepare vegetables to reap the most nutritive value out of them? There is good value in eating vegetables raw, but in fact lightly steamed vegetables may be better for you. Depending on the vegetable, raw forms provide limited nutrients, and their primary benefit may be the fiber alone. Light steaming breaks down the cell walls and makes the phytonutrients better absorbed within your cells. These phytonutrients are compounds in plants that can bolster our defenses against agents of disease, reducing risks of cancer and other serious illnesses.

As an example, raw carrots are virtually free of calories, and their nutrients are virtually unavailable; cooked or juiced carrots, however, contribute calories as well as a host of valuable phytonutrients. Cooking and juicing also releases a lot of flavor in the carrot, changing the taste from somewhat bland to very sweet (not recommended for diabetics). Juicing is equivalent to cooking in releasing phytonutrients because the blades of the juicer break down the cell walls by mechanical means. Juicing eliminates the fiber, however, and in the case of foods such as carrots, beets, or apples, results in something that may be nutrient rich but off the glycemic index chart. Chewing slowly and thoroughly is also an effective way to release the nutrients. This is a healthful practice for all foods you consume.

3. Choose the right oils to maximize your intake of healthy "good" fats versus unhealthy "bad" fats.

There are good fats, bad fats, and really bad fats. Saturated fats are bad fats that are found in animal meat and dairy products. Unsaturated fats are either monounsaturated or polyunsaturated. Both are good fats that come from various plant, nut, and fish oil sources that remain liquid at room temperature. Last, there are "trans fats," or trans-fatty acids, that are *really bad* fats, also known as partially hydrogenated fats. This last type was created by the food-processing companies in their quest to extend the shelf life of processed foods by simulating polyunsaturated fat that remains solid at room temperature.

You may hold the assumption that the higher your fat intake, the more risk you have for developing cardiovascular disease. The fact is that as you consume higher levels of saturated fats, such as red meat and dairy products, your cardiovascular risk becomes greater, as these fats raise cholesterol levels, especially LDL, the "bad" cholesterol. However, consuming certain unsaturated fats can actually *lower* your cardiovascular risk, by helping promote a healthy ratio of HDL levels (good cholesterol) to LDL levels (bad cholesterol).

Residents of Mediterranean countries such as Greece and Italy have a diet high in cold-pressed olive oil, fresh fruits and vegetables, and fish instead of red meat. Almost every meal features a dish fried, sautéed, or tossed in olive oil; yet Mediterranean countries report low rates of cardiovascular disease.

Based on this medical evidence, you are making a healthy choice when you use quality extra-virgin olive oil for a wide range of your culinary needs. Quality extra-virgin olive oil is unrefined and cold pressed. No heat is used in extracting the oil from the olives, preserving its nutrients.

On the other hand, other vegetable oils go through more extensive processing in which heat is used to increase oil yields. Adding heat to oils oxidizes them and destroys the nutrients; oils that ordinarily are good for you are transformed at high temperatures into sources of harmful free radicals that accelerate aging.

The ideal salad dressing base includes organic expeller-pressed extra-virgin olive oil with balsamic vinegar or unsweetened rice vinegar. For cooking, your best option is olive oil, which holds together at moderately high temperatures and resists oxidation much better than other vegetable oils.

No discussion of good and bad fats would be complete without taking a stand in the margarine versus butter controversy. The reason this controversy never seems to disappear completely is probably due to the fact that both butter and margarine are bad for you. Even taking into account its high saturated fat content, organic butter might be considered "healthier" as it contains no trans-fatty acids or hydrogenated fats.

Hydrogenated fats, copiously present in margarine and vegetable shortening, are the worst kind of fats you can eat. To hydrogenate oil, manufacturers heat the oil at extremely high temperatures with hydrogen gas in nickel or platinum catalysts for several hours. This process destroys the oil's chemical structure and converts it into damaged polyunsaturated fat called trans-fatty acids, or TFAs.

Your cell membranes, which control the transport of fats in and out of the cell, are thoroughly confused when TFAs are present. When they are put into the cell membrane, the membrane gets stiff and does not function properly. TFAs create similar havoc in the fat layer of your cells that must be replenished and maintained to preserve the cell's integrity.

Hydrogenated and partially hydrogenated fats are a dangerous component of margarine and other food products. Read the labels of the brands of peanut butter, crackers, and other foods you have purchased recently to see this for yourself. These dangerous fats were designed to extend shelf life and to remain solid throughout a wide temperature range; this prevents the oils in your margarine and peanut butter from liquefying and separating at room temperature. This cosmetic improvement in the appearance of these products has come at a grave cost: a growing incidence of hardening of the arteries among millions of adults today.

Regarding the three natural types of oils and fats—saturated, monounsaturated, and polyunsaturated—it is important to eliminate saturated fats from your diet and moderately consume monounsaturated and polyunsaturated fats, as they all are highly caloric. The list below provides a breakdown of each type.

FATS AND OILS

Saturated Fats/Oils	Monounsaturated Oils	Polyunsaturated Oils
Animal fat	Avocado oil	Corn oil
Butterfat	Olive oil	Cottonseed oil
Coconut oil	Peanut oil	Fish oil
Palm kernel oil		Flaxseed oil
Palm oil		Grapeseed oil
		Safflower oil
		Sesame oil
		Soybean oil
		Sunflower oil
		Walnut oil

Essential Fatty Acids: Omega-3 and Omega-6

Most foods that contain fat typically comprise a blend of two or all three types of fats. At least 30 percent of your fat intake should include polyunsaturated oils, as they provide the two essential fats required by your body to maintain cellular health: the linoleic acid family (omega-6), and the alpha-linolenic acid family (omega-3). The ideal balance between these two is about twice as much omega-6 as omega-3. Most people are deficient in omega-3 fats and obtain more omega-6 fats than necessary from their foods. A high intake of saturated fats and TFAs precludes the body from making good use of the small quantity of essential fats the average person consumes in a day.

Omega-6 fats are converted into gamma-linolenic acid (GLA), dihomo gamma-linolenic acid (DGLA), and then into series 1 prostaglandins. These prostaglandins keep the blood thin, prevent clots and blockages, relax blood vessels, lower blood pressure, improve nerve and immune function, and help insulin work more efficiently to help balance blood sugar. Good sources of GLA are evening primrose oil (1,500 mg a day) or borage oil (750 mg a day).

Omega-3 fats, which often need to be supplemented, are essential for proper brain function and affect vision, learning ability, coordination, and mood. These essential fats also reduce inflammation (beneficial for arthritis, lupus, and other inflammatory diseases), control cholesterol, and improve immune function as well as metabolism. The best sources of omega-3 fats are seed oils and carnivorous fish. The best seed oils for omega-3 fats are flax (also known as linseed), hemp, walnut, and pumpkin. The best fish include mackerel, herring, and salmon. An optimal intake would be one 1,000 mg capsule two times a day or one-half to one tablespoon of oil a day, or one to two tablespoons of ground flaxseeds, or a six-ounce serving of a fish listed above.

4. Optimize your fiber intake. Eat a variety of whole grains and legumes (peas, beans, and lentils), as well as fresh fruits and vegetables.

We have already detailed the benefits of whole grains, legumes, fruits, and vegetables as a carbohydrate source. Additionally, they offer an important dietary source of fiber that is essential for intestinal health and eliminating toxins. In a variety of whole foods, from grains and legumes to fruits and vegetables, a high proportion of the nutrients are present in or just beneath the skin or husk. In grains, the outer covering is called the bran.

A grain is whole and unrefined if the entire kernel is left unaltered and intact. There are three parts to a whole grain:

the endosperm (containing mostly starch and protein), germ (rich in unsaturated fats, protein, carbohydrates, vitamin E, B complex vitamins, and minerals), and bran (containing a large density of fiber, minerals, and B vitamins). During refining, the most nutritional part of the grain (the germ and bran) is removed (including plant sterols that are helpful in disease prevention), leaving only the endosperm.

Most of the grains found in supermarket breads and cereals are refined for greater marketability. Additionally, sugar or other sweeteners are added to most of these products, making them even less healthy. For optimum nutritional value, it is best to purchase sprouted, whole-grain bread, tortillas, and bagels. Also, whole oats offer significant nutritional value versus oatmeal or rolled oats; if it is instant or cooks in less than ten minutes, it is not very nutritious.

Just because a product label boasts "whole grain" it does not guarantee good nutrition. Look for a whole-grain product as the first ingredient on the list. The best whole-grain products include whole wheat, oats, amaranth, barley, buckwheat, and millet. If the food is described as cracked wheat, multigrain, oat bran, whole bran, wheat berry, rye bread, or seven or nine grain, you are looking at mostly refined (processed) grains. When choosing grains, organic is best; for flours, select only whole-grain or stone-ground, whole-wheat, unbleached varieties. If you have a wheat allergy, choose gluten-free products.

When selecting rice, you have the choice of white rice in which the bran has been removed, or brown rice, in which the bran is intact. White rice was developed in China, the first country to remove the bran layer from brown rice. The Chinese aristocracy preferred white over brown rice, finding it to be much more elegant; however, they started dying from a B vitamin deficiency and eventually returned to eating brown rice.

You may never have heard of quinoa (pronounced keen-wah), but this so-called grain (it is technically a fruit) deserves to be singled out here for its unique properties. Quinoa has been grown and consumed in high-altitude regions of Latin America for five thousand years. Available at most health food stores, quinoa contains 16 percent protein and high amounts of essential fatty acids. This is a much higher percent of protein than most grains. It is also a solid source of vitamins and minerals, including calcium, vitamin E, iron, and B vitamins. You can use quinoa for a high-protein change of pace in any recipe that calls for rice. It is excellent served cold or hot.

Legumes consist of chickpeas, soybeans, black beans, black-eyed peas, kidney beans, and lentils, among others. These are all excellent sources of fiber provided the cooking method preserves the nutrient value. As with cooking vegetables, to maintain nutrients and fiber integrity never overcook legumes.

5. Find your hidden sources of refined sugar and eliminate it from your diet; employ a healthy alternative when you feel the need to sweeten foods.

Refined sugar is present in the vast majority of processed food products available in supermarkets today and often hides behind an alias such as glucose, fructose, sucrose, dextrose, maltose, or corn syrup. Rather than allowing consumers to experience the natural flavors of foods, food-processing companies add an unhealthy sweetener to almost every product. As a natural result of this pervasive proliferation of sugar, rates of diabetes are rising all over the world.

In countless studies, sugar has been blamed for more than diabetes. It contributes to hyperactivity, attention deficit disorder, severe mood swings, decreased brain function, serious digestive problems, yeast infections, obesity, and tooth decay. It also depletes your body of B vitamins and leaches calcium from your hair, bones, blood, and teeth. It interferes with the absorption of calcium, protein, and other important minerals in the body. Sugar also retards the growth of valuable intestinal bacteria and inhibits the secretion of gastric juices, impeding digestion. It also seriously inhibits the immune system. All in all, sugar is one of the most serious robbers of health.

You need not participate in this excess sugar consumption; you can take action to protect yourself and your family from diabetes and insulin resistance. Eliminate refined sugar, and do not replace it with carcinogenic chemical sugar substitutes such as saccharine and aspartame. Here are some good alternatives to white and brown sugar:

- **Xylitol.** Xylitol is a natural product obtained from the birch tree, without sugar's harmful side effects. Xylitol can be found in a granulated form that looks and tastes like sugar, and can be substituted measure for measure (1:1).

- **Stevia.** Stevia is a natural plant-based sweetener. One advantage to stevia is that it is naturally so sweet that you do not need to use very much of it.

- **Pure honey, pure maple syrup, or pure maple sugar.** The caveat with using these substitutes is that people tend to ladle them on, until their food is literally swimming in a lake of honey or syrup. To avoid adverse health consequences, use these substitutes sparingly. Additionally, diabetics should avoid these forms of sweeteners altogether.

6. Incorporate foods representing "colors of the rainbow" at every meal.

Each color present in vegetables and fruits supplies a different mix of vitamins, minerals, phytonutrients, and antioxidants. Dark, rich colors are often an indicator of higher levels of nutrients. For example, the typical American salad is primarily comprised of iceberg lettuce, which has virtually no nutritional value. To optimize your health, enjoy a large salad every day including mixed spring lettuce, spinach, or other dark green leafy lettuce, mixed with bell peppers (red, yellow, orange, and/or green), cucumbers, blanched broccoli and/or asparagus, carrots, and avocado (in moderation), as well as tomatoes or other fruits and vegetables of choice to provide optimum levels of phytonutrients needed by your body.

Keep this "color of the rainbow" concept in mind when preparing your meals. For a complete balanced meal, add walnuts or raw sunflower seeds and broiled salmon or chicken to your salad. Remember, the more natural and colorful the foods, the healthier the meal.

7. Consume at least two quarts of water per day to keep your body hydrated for optimal health. Minimize or avoid alcoholic, caffeinated, and carbonated beverages that have dehydrating properties and leach vitamins and minerals from your body.

Since your body is two-thirds water, it is not surprising that water is one of the most important nutrients for good health.

Your body uses at least one quart of water a day to excrete toxins and impurities in the form of sweat, breath vapor, and urine. To keep your natural detoxification processes running efficiently, you should consume at least two quarts of filtered or purified water a day. Herbal teas such as peppermint or chamomile can be counted as water, but not sodas, coffee, or juices.

Depending on where you live, the amount of impurities in the water supply can vary widely. Chlorine, toxic chemicals, and heavy metals can be present in tap water. You can purchase bottled water or install a water filter. Filters are available to remove impurities and chemicals; you can attach a filter directly to your faucet or pass water through a filter attached to a pitcher. If you choose to use filters, closely follow the manufacturer's recommendations for filter replacement. After two to six months, filters lose most of their effectiveness.

Most of us drink a variety of beverages, not just water. In this aspect of nutrition, as in so many others, there are unhealthful choices and more healthful ones. Some beverages are powerful diuretics, causing you to urinate more frequently and contributing to dehydration. Explore the advantages and disadvantages of your favorite beverages in the following table.

BEVERAGES PROS AND CONS

Beverage	Pros	Cons	Notes
Sodas/soft drinks	None	Contain sugar and/or artificial sweeteners, as well as chemicals. Carbonation and high levels of phosphorus leach minerals, such as calcium and magnesium, out of your body.	All types of soda are bad for you whether caffeine free or diet.
Carbonated drinks		Carbonation and high levels of phosphorus both leach minerals, such as calcium and magnesium, out of your body.	Naturally carbonated drinks are fine, but there are very few naturally carbonated beverages available.
Coffee	Some antioxidants are present in coffee that is served and consumed fresh.	High levels of caffeine, diuretic properties.	Should be consumed fresh (within twenty minutes of making it). If drinking decaf, choose water-process decaffeinated; other varieties use formaldehyde to remove the caffeine.
Tea, herbal	Contains antioxidants, and does not contain caffeine.	None	Unlike coffee, tea retains its antioxidant benefits even when it is not fresh.

BEVERAGES PROS AND CONS (Continued)

Beverage	Pros	Cons	Notes
Tea, green or black	Green tea and black tea both supply antioxidants, polyphenols, and corsitin.	Most contain caffeine.	Unlike coffee, tea retains its antioxidant benefits even when it is not fresh.
Hard alcohol and beer	None	Diuretic properties, contains toxins.	Consumption of more than three glasses daily may cause liver damage.
Fruit juices	100 percent natural all-fruit juices provide a source of vitamin C.	High concentration of fructose (natural sugar).	Dilute juice with water (50/50).
Juice drinks	May provide a source of vitamin C.	High concentration of fructose (natural sugar) and many add refined sugar.	Not recommended.
Wine	Contains antioxidants and polyphenols.	Diuretic properties, contains toxins.	Red wine contains more antioxidants than white wine. Consumption of more than three glasses daily may cause liver damage.

8. Eat raw or dry roasted seeds and nuts (not ones roasted with oil).

Seeds and nuts are an excellent source of protein and good fats. However, roasting nuts and seeds using heat and oil destroys the natural protein and vitamins, increases sugar levels, and oxidizes fats.

The table below compares the nutritional value of common nut and seed varieties.

1 Cup Seeds/Nuts	Total Calories	Total Fat	Saturated Fat (Bad)	Poly-unsaturated fat	Mono-unsaturated fat	Protein
Almonds*	549 kcal	48.1 g	3.7 g	11.6 g	30.5 g	20.2 g
Brazil nuts	918 kcal	92.7 g	22.6 g	33.8 g	32.2 g	20.1 g
Cashews (dry roasted, no salt added)	786 kcal	63.5 g	12.5 g	10.7 g	37.4 g	21 g
Macadamia Nuts (raw)	962 kcal	101.5 g	16.2 g	2 g	78.9 g	10.6 g
Peanuts	827 kcal	71.9 g	10 g	22.7 g	35.7 g	37.7 g
Pecans* (dry roasted, unsalted)	201 kcal	21.1 g	1.8 g	5.8 g	12.5 g	2.7 g
Pine nuts (dried)*	768 kcal	69 g	10.6 g	29 g	25.9 g	32.6 g
Pistachio nuts (raw)	705 kcal	55.3 g	6.8 g	16.7 g	29 g	26.2 g
Pumpkin seeds* (dry, unsalted)	746 kcal	63.3 g	12 g	28.8 g	19.7 g	33.9 g
Sesame seeds*	825 kcal	71.5 g	10 g	31.4 g	27 g	25.5 g
Sunflower Seeds* (dry, unsalted)	745 kcal	63.7 g	6.7 g	42.1 g	12.2 g	24.7 g
Walnuts*	784 kcal	78.3 g	7.4 g	56.6 g	10.7 g	18.3 g

* Denotes the healthiest nuts/seeds to consume in moderation.

When purchasing nut butters, such as almond butter, scrutinize the label carefully. Many varieties are full of undesirable ingredients added during processing, such as salt, sugar, and hydrogenated and partially hydrogenated fats. Varieties made with raw nuts to which nothing has been added are the most nutritious. Nut butters need to be refrigerated to avoid oil separation.

9. Minimize your consumption of processed foods.

Processed foods are those that are prepackaged, refined, and ultimately nutrient deficient. Unfortunately, due to the element of convenience and perceived lack of time to prepare whole nutritious foods, processed foods are now considered a staple in the average household. Without regard for the detrimental impact processed foods have on our health, the consumption of these convenience foods has skyrocketed over the past few decades. An entire industry has arisen that profits at the expense of our health.

Adults have choices about what they eat—young children do not. They typically have to eat what they are served. Unfortunately, too many parents are feeding their children foods that contain carcinogenic chemicals, dyes, and preservatives, without realizing the consequences.

Minimize the amount of processed foods purchased for home consumption. You and your family may be forced to eat processed foods when you are at work, school, and traveling on vacation or business. Why expose yourself and your family to the guaranteed health risks of processed foods when you have control over the foods you eat at home?

Although these are less convenient than processed foods, you will reap tremendous health benefits by stocking your pantry and refrigerator with fresh fruits, vegetables, beans, whole grains, fish, and poultry. As described throughout this chapter, there are many health benefits to eating well-balanced, nutritious meals.

10. When you have the luxury of eating at home, maximize the control you have over your food choices and prepare for being away.

Engaging in healthy habits over an extended period at home builds up your reserves. This gives you an extra margin of protection against depleting your reserves when business or vacation takes you out of town.

If you do not arm yourself with healthy alternatives, you are at the mercy of what the road has to offer. You may find yourself stuck for several days in an unfamiliar city where the only food choices seem to be fast-food restaurants or unhealthy vending machine selections. How can you take control of what you eat? When traveling, you can stay in total control of your diet and health by carrying a snack pack of nutritious foods at all times and replenishing it as needed at a local grocery store.

The best option is a small cooler or insulated container. To keep the foods in your snack pack fresh for the long haul, freeze a bottle or two of drinking water and place it in the bottom, then stack your food on top. As the frozen water begins to melt, you can drink it to fulfill your daily water consumption requirement.

Chapter Summary

The topic of good nutrition is both complex and extensive. It has been studied for centuries and has been proven to contribute to optimum health and vitality. Medical evidence points to countless physical and mental diseases that are a result of poor nutrition; conversely, good health and vitality has been linked to optimum nutrition.

To make food a healing force rather than a destructive one, at every meal it is important to consume the recommended ratio of protein, carbohydrates, and "good" fats, as described throughout this chapter. Consume food wisely and mindfully, as food is medicine. Follow the ten recommendations below and eat your way to optimized health and vitality.

Ten Practical Ways to Eat Balanced, Nutritious Meals

1. Optimize your protein intake. Virtually eliminate red meat and animal fats from your diet; instead consume fish, poultry, and plant sources of protein (soy beans, legumes, nuts, and grains).
2. Optimize your carbohydrate intake. Eat fresh organic fruits and vegetables, as well as whole grains and beans.
3. Optimize your fat intake. Choose the right oils to maximize your intake of healthy "good" fats versus unhealthy "bad" fats.
4. Optimize your fiber intake. Eat a variety of whole grains and legumes (peas, beans, and lentils), as well as fresh fruits and vegetables.
5. Find your hidden sources of sugar and eliminate it from your diet; employ a healthy alternative when you feel the need to sweeten foods.

6. Incorporate foods representing "colors of the rainbow" at every meal.

7. Consume at least two quarts of water per day to keep your body hydrated for optimal health. Minimize or avoid alcoholic, caffeinated, and carbonated beverages that have dehydrating properties and leach vitamins and minerals from your body.

8. Eat raw or dry roasted seeds and nuts (not ones roasted with oil).

9. Minimize your consumption of processed foods.

10. When you have the luxury of eating at home, maximize the control you have over your food choices and prepare for being away.

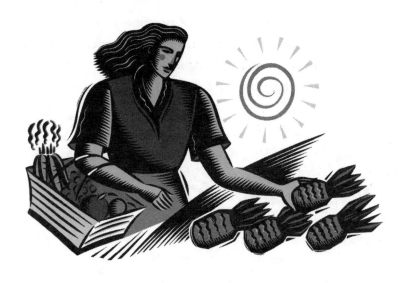

Taking the time to optimize your kitchen for preparing nutri-

tious meals is the foundation of healthy eating.

Key Factor Five
Perform a Healthy Kitchen Makeover

When you consider all the rooms of a house, the kitchen is really the center of the home. It is a place where you find warmth, comfort, and a neutral ground for open interactions. It is the one common room where everyone is welcome without an invitation. When I was growing up, we typically shared our opinions and thoughts and discussed our day's events over family meals.

For us, as is true with most families, the refrigerator, pantry, and cupboards were open territory. We were able to eat or drink just about anything that was in the kitchen. Instead of fresh fruits and vegetables when I needed a snack, I would naturally opt for foods that conveniently came out of a box or bag. Having had an addiction to all of the traditional junk foods, and in order to eliminate the temptation of eating these damaging foods, I had to do a complete healthy kitchen makeover. I found that to make it as easy as possible to maintain a healthful diet, it would be important to control what foods I stocked in my kitchen.

The ten practical ways to conduct a healthy kitchen makeover outlined in this chapter will give you a clear sense of how to take the first steps to make cooking healthful foods easy and fun.

—Jodi L. Jones

In Western civilization, we have some truly odd ideas and practices regarding food and cooking. A keen observer might even conclude that we have a dysfunctional relationship with food. We use food as a reward, and even sometimes as punishment; we use it to give ourselves pleasure and comfort, and we use it to fill our emotional voids.

Food can be your friend or your enemy. This chapter will discuss how to have a lifelong healthy friendship with food—one that will be forged inside the walls and cabinets of your kitchen.

Most Americans are very fortunate to be able to purchase and eat whatever we want and to choose what we eat and how it will be prepared. In many countries, people are starving and must eat whatever they can find. More often than not, what is available is not fresh, healthy, or nutritionally adequate. We are spoiled by an abundance of beautiful food and healthy possibilities.

Motivating Your Family and Yourself

When it comes to eating healthy food, nothing is a more effective motivator than a serious medical condition. The right foods can really make a big difference in reducing symptoms of grave conditions such as diabetes, arthritis, or even cancer. But it should not take this kind of dire threat to your health to bring every member of your family on board with your new eating plan.

It is not at all uncommon to exhibit symptoms that can be improved by healthy eating or a combination of improved diet and nutritional supplements. If your family members suffer from acne, allergies, fatigue, asthma, headaches, mood swings, or digestive problems, they may be more than willing to join you in this quest for good health—especially if they understand the connection between nutrition and health.

Your feelings about food, and the origins of the dysfunctional relationship you may have with your food, most certainly came, at least in part, from messages your parents gave you about food at an early age. For generations, parents have been conveying uneducated messages about nutrition and diet, messages that place the wrong value on foods. A comment parents typically make to their children is, "Eat all your vegetables and you can have ice cream." The message here is that vegetables do not taste good and have to be choked down and that ice cream is much better than vegetables.

Do not fall into the trap of rewarding children (or yourself) with food, especially when the reward is bad for them (and you). Take rewards out of the equation entirely. Serve your children one of the healthy dessert recipes you will find in Appendix E of this book as a normal part of a complete and healthy meal. This way they will enjoy dessert but not see it as a reward.

Financial Ramifications of Healthy Eating

Overall, there is no need to spend more money than usual on food when transitioning to the kind of healthful diet we describe in this book. Few things in a supermarket carry higher price tags than processed cereals, candy, sodas, snack foods, and desserts. You will discover that nutritious high-fiber food is more filling, and that you will eat smaller portions, which can also cut down on your food costs. The money you save will amount to more than enough to pay the slight cost difference between organic and nonorganic foods. Do not forget that fast food can also be quite expensive, especially when you buy it several times per week.

Some Thoughts on Eating Out

Very few people have the discipline to adhere to a healthy regimen for three meals a day, seven days a week, without deviation, especially when they are away from home. The idea is to be firm when you are at home, when you have control over your kitchen environment and your ingredients. As you learn which ingredients are healthful and which are health destroying, you will be more informed and make smarter choices on the meals you eat away from home.

There is nothing wrong with rewarding yourself for your commitment to this program by treating yourself to a meal out at your favorite restaurant. But even when you are eating out, there is a healthy approach and an unhealthy one. For example, when having a Mexican meal out, focus on that lobster enchilada you've been dreaming about and do not fill up on the unhealthy appetizers and grease-laden fried tortilla chips that you can easily live without. Indulge, but only fill yourself with your favorite foods, ones that are really worth it.

When you go to a restaurant, plan beforehand what you are going to eat, what you are going to skip, and how much you will need to eat to feel pleasurably filled without being stuffed. You should also consider bringing your own healthy salad dressing and whole-wheat crackers so you are not so tempted to indulge in the unhealthy choices typically available at most restaurants.

Choose restaurant meals not from the perspective of losing weight, but from the perspective of overall health. People tend to make choices based on what is more fattening, instead of what the physiological impact will be when they ingest ingredients into their bodies. Ask yourself, how is my body going to be able to assimilate this? Which choices are going to give me the most energy, the most nourishment for my brain, and make me feel the best when I go to sleep? What will make me feel bloated and uncomfortable?

Read on for the ten recommendations for a healthy kitchen. Change may not come easily at first, but the rewards will be great; the health of your family is at stake. Be sure to adhere to these recommendations very closely when at home, because it will be all the more difficult to observe them when you are away.

Ten Practical Ways to Perform a Healthy Kitchen Makeover

1. Invest in quality tools to make cooking easier. Organize your kitchen to make accessing these tools convenient.

Not having the right tools close at hand just makes cooking more difficult and more of a chore. Quality tools can really cut your preparation time dramatically and increase the pleasure you derive from cooking.

Below is a list of tools you will need to cook nutritious meals efficiently:

- Knives—chef's knife, utility knife, and tomato knife (stainless steel or carbon steel)

- Knife sharpener
- Vegetable brush
- Electric steamer (a combination food steamer and rice steamer is ideal)
- Pots and pans—buy stainless steel, stoneware, or Pyrex/ glass cookware; avoid aluminum or aluminum coated (aluminum's soft texture can cause toxic elements to leach into the food), and cast iron. If you cook anything in cast iron that is mildly acidic, it will add iron to the food. Iron is an oxidizing agent, the most common nutritional excess in our country, and can easily be toxic to children. Additionally, unless you know how to properly care for and season cast iron, it will rust easily.
- Large soup (stock) pot
- Food processor
- Small electric chopper
- Blender
- Small coffee bean grinder (for finely grinding flaxseeds)
- Fine strainer for rinsing rice and a colander for draining pasta
- Vegetable slicer, garlic press, apple corer, chopper
- Various colored chopping mats (separate color for meats, vegetables, fruits, and fish)
- Water purification system

When using a microwave, we recommend that you use it to simply reheat foods or boil water. Do not heat foods, especially those containing fat, in plastic containers, and do not cover foods with plastic wrap. The combination of high heat, fat, and plastic releases dioxins into the food, which can ultimately leach into the cells of our bodies. Dioxins are carcinogens and are highly toxic to our cells. Instead, heat your food in glass or ceramic containers, and cover your food with paper towels.

2. Inventory your pantry, refrigerator, freezer, and cupboards and donate (or eliminate) any unhealthful foods you find lurking in your house or apartment.

The concept here is that if you do not have immediate access to unhealthy foods and ingredients, you will not be nearly as tempted to consume them. What you do not have, you cannot eat.

If your family is typical, your shelves, cupboards, and refrigerator are overflowing with bags, cans, and boxes of processed foods, candy, soda, white flour–based breads and crackers, sugar-based foods and cereals, ice cream, and so on. Read the labels on some of these packages and educate yourself about the unhealthful ingredients in some of your favorite foods; they are probably full of sugar, hydrogenated fats, preservatives, chemicals, and other antinutrients that you should avoid in the interest of optimizing your health.

The temptation to stray from nutritious choices is especially powerful when you are eating away from home, so keep your kitchen healthy so that you can stay strong and resist temptation when you are at home. After a couple of weeks of instituting more healthy eating choices, you will not really miss the unhealthy foods and empty calories.

The most effective strategy here is to make the change all at one time. For many, however, it may be more realistic to create a transition plan by preparing your family for the changes that lie ahead in the refrigerator, freezer, and pantry. Start by substituting snack foods the first week, then breakfast foods the second, moving to lunch during the third week, then dinner the fourth.

Over the course of this month of transition, try not to feel bad about depriving your family members of their favorite, unwholesome foods. You will be surprised at how well they survive and make the adjustment, and you will be giving your spouse and children the gift of a lifetime of healthy nutritional habits. To undo the effects of years of unhealthy eating habits, your children may need a little tough love; go cold turkey by completely eliminating unhealthful food items in your pantry and kitchen all at once.

3. Replace the processed foods you disposed of during your kitchen makeover with fresh whole foods.

Stock quality fresh and prepared spices, fresh fruits and vegetables, whole grains, filtered water, green tea, plain non-fat yogurt, raw nuts and seeds, whole (steel-cut) oats, and so on. Whole foods are far richer than processed foods in vitality, flavor, fiber, and phytonutrients.

As for herbs and spices, it is not realistic to assume that you will have access to fresh herbs every day of the year, even if you have an organic garden in your backyard. Therefore, you will need to acquire and rely on some bottled spices and spice mixes. Blended organic spices, containing several to as many as a dozen kinds of dried herbs, can be an excellent solution to add flavor to your recipes quickly and easily. Instead of pulling out a dozen different spice bottles and shaking out a few pinches of each, you can just shake out a teaspoon or two from one bottle. Read the labels here as well; organic, salt-free blends are the most healthful.

4. Plan your menus weekly to maximize variety and vitality in your diet. Make sure to complete your weekly menu plan before you go out to shop for food.

Focus on balanced meals when planning your weekly menus. Every meal should contain a balanced mix of protein, beneficial fats, and carbohydrates. For most healthy people, the ideal balanced meal consists of 15 percent protein, 15 percent wholesome fats, and 70 percent carbohydrates. For overweight people and those with low blood sugar, 30 percent protein, 30 percent healthy fats, and 40 percent carbohydrates is the ideal balance. These percentages vary based on specific health conditions and health goals. It is best to consult your nutritional medical practitioner for a personalized plan.

By maintaining a three-ring binder containing your favorite healthy recipes for breakfast, lunch, dinner, desserts, appetizers, and side dishes, you will always have the information you need for effective planning close at hand. Decide in advance which days you will eat together as a family, and which days you must eat out, and commit to the schedule.

You will save time and money if you always do the meal plan before you go out shopping. You may find that you are doing much of this preshopping planning already. Preparing for healthier meals may not take any more time than you are currently spending on this process.

The act of planning and cooking nutritious meals every day is one of the most important things you can do for your family. When you find yourself frequently putting social, school, and work commitments ahead of this critical activity, you are shortchanging your family and yourself. No matter how busy your schedule, you have to make the time.

5. When cooking, make extra of each item for leftovers to use throughout the rest of the week.

The goal in menu planning is to maximize both variety and convenience. You can accomplish this by making large quantities of staple foods one day (brown rice, beans, chicken, and so on), then making creative combinations with those staples on subsequent days.

You may discover that it works best for you to set aside a large block of time on the weekend to cook basics for the rest of the week (chicken broth, brown rice, couscous, chicken, and so on). Some cooks spend as many as four to six hours one day a week, but find that the extra time they gain during the week more than makes up for this commitment.

By preparing ahead of time all the staple foods that take more than an hour to cook, you can cut about half an hour off your cooking time every night. Add fresh ingredients when using leftovers to add variety and vitality to the meal. Use this opportunity to prepare healthy lunches for the next day for you and your family.

Leftover quantities of chicken can be used as the base for salads, soups, a brown rice casserole, whole-wheat pizza, and chicken roll-ups. The table on page 129 lists some common staple foods and shows how you can reuse each food throughout the week. You will save a lot of time and effort with this strategy.

Another money-saving strategy is to spend five minutes a day examining your refrigerator and cabinets for foods that are about to expire. Do not let food go bad. Freeze it, puree it, or share it with friends and neighbors. Why waste money?

6. Make cooking fun and social—invite a friend to cook with you, or make cooking a family event and include lots of fun for the kids.

For some of us, cooking has never been that much fun and is regarded as a chore. Many of our attitudes about cooking are developed at an early age based on our family situation. Perhaps this activity was forced on you as one of your daily chores and not positioned as a "family bonding" activity.

If this describes your experiences with cooking, you should take the opportunity to make cooking more pleasurable by making it a social occasion. Recruiting a neighbor or friend to become your cooking buddy can really take the drudgery out of shopping and cooking. You can exchange recipes and learn from each other about a variety of new techniques and cuisines. You can share expenses and cook double portions for both your families, and you will receive 100 percent of the personal rewards and appreciation from your family in exchange for only 50 percent of the work. You will spend much less time at the market, too, since you will only be making half as many trips to the store as you did before.

Cooking as a family represents a golden opportunity to educate your children and instill values about good nutrition very early in life. Children love to help with the hand work, and you can choose tasks where they will not be endangered by sharp or dangerous tools, such as mashing potatoes, taking peas out of the pods, shelling nuts, shredding chicken by hand, or washing mushrooms with a vegetable brush. If your kids are old enough to handle it, buy them a mini-chopper (less hazardous than a food processor) and set up a separate station in the kitchen for them where they can help Mom or Dad prepare the meal.

Set a good and healthy example for your children to follow. Daughters always want to learn how to do whatever mom is doing. When Dad is doing the cooking, your son will want to help out. Fathers can be great role models for teaching their sons to be comfortable and handy around the kitchen.

7. Do not feel obliged to make everything from scratch. Use quality prepared food items when necessary.

You may be surprised to discover the wide range of basic whole foods that are available in your neighborhood supermarket. Whole grains and dried beans are readily available, for example, and can form the basis for a natural foods meal that will not entail a separate shopping trip to a specialty store.

Some ingredients may be a little harder to come by. You will find recipes for making black beans, tzatziki, hummus, low-sodium organic broth, and other staples from scratch in this book (see Appendix E); however, in a pinch, feel free to use quality prepared foods found in farmers' markets or health food stores.

When shopping for quality prepared foods, be sure to scrutinize the labels carefully to ensure that the item doesn't contain preservatives, sugar (in its many forms), hydrogenated or partially hydrogenated fats, white flour, or chemical ingredients with so many syllables you cannot even pronounce them.

8. Listen to soothing music or watch a relaxing TV show as "background" if cooking alone. Do not watch anything distressing or distracting.

Good food preparation demands a relaxed and motivated state of mind, especially if you do not like to cook. You have to do whatever puts you in the mood and will make you feel good about making a nutritious meal. The right frame of mind makes cooking a treat, not a chore.

The key is finding out what works best for you. It may sound a little extreme, but some people find that their optimal time to cook is at 10 P.M., after the kids have gone to bed. They have the house all to themselves, they can put on their favorite music, and they do not have the kids running around, making noise, demanding attention, and creating distractions. At that time, you can cook all the meals and lunches for the next day. As dinnertime approaches, all you will have to do is warm up the food and serve it. The pressure will be off, and you will be able to serve the meal in minutes.

9. Create or try a new recipe each week to keep a little spice in your life.

Buy new healthy cookbooks—they can be a great source

for new recipes and cooking ideas. Also, read magazines that contain healthy recipes. When you find one that contains a couple of your favorite ingredients, give it a try.

When picking out a recipe to test, bear in mind that recipes do not need to be complex—in fact, the simpler the better. Obviously, simpler recipes can also be made more quickly. In general, look for recipes that have fewer than ten ingredients. The length of the recipe instructions is another factor to consider. If it takes four pages to describe how to make the recipe, it might be too complicated and demotivating for most nonprofessional cooks. When it comes to healthy recipes and cookbooks, look for words such as "healthy" and "nutritious," along with "quick" and "easy" featured prominently on the cover.

The best way to build up your recipe library is to skim quickly through recipe books, marking each interesting one with a note. Photocopy all the pages that interest you and put those pages in a three-ring binder. You will never have to pore through a stack of cookbooks again looking for something new to try, because you will have gathered all your promising prospects for healthy dishes in one convenient place.

After you have prepared the recipe, make a few notes on the page in your binder. Jot down if your family enjoyed it, what substitutions you would make in ingredients, and what changes you would make in preparation. The dish will turn out even better the next time you serve it.

A final word of advice is to be creative and experiment in the kitchen—do not always accept recipes as "literal." As your cooking experience grows, you will become aware of which ingredients taste good together, and which ingredients your family is less than enthusiastic about seeing included in a meal. One sure sign of a good cook is the ability to rummage around in a refrigerator and pantry, choose a few simple ingredients, and combine them into a healthful, delicious meal—without ever looking at a recipe card.

10. Rewrite all your favorite unhealthy recipes. You can transform each one into a much more healthful recipe by substituting selected ingredients.

The chapter on nutrition will inform you of the reasoning behind making these substitutions. To create more healthy meals, substitute the ingredients on the left with the more nutritious choices from the column on the right.

FOOD SUBSTITUTES

Substitute	With
White flour	Whole-wheat or brown rice flour
Refined white or brown sugar	Xylitol, Stevia, maple sugar, unfiltered honey, rice syrup
Milk	Soy milk, rice milk, or multigrain nondairy drink
Margarine or butter	Extra-virgin olive oil, grape seed oil, avocado oil, or other healthy oil (if you must have butter, use organic ghee or clarified butter)
Beef stock	Homemade roasted chicken, turkey, or vegetable stock
White rice	Brown rice or cous cous
Canned fruits and vegetables	Fresh organic fruits and vegetables
Chips and snacks	Whole-wheat sesame crackers with hummus, stone-ground whole-wheat crackers with natural peanut butter

Peanut butter (with added hydrogenated or partially hydrogenated fats and added sugar) and jelly (with added sugar) on white bread	Natural organic peanut butter (or other raw nut butter) and pure fruit spread on sprouted whole-wheat toast
Donut, egg bagel, or white salted bagel with cream cheese	Whole-wheat sprouted bagel with pure fruit spread
Mayonnaise	Soy-based sandwich spread or plain yogurt
Coffee	Decaffeinated green tea and other herbal teas
Sodas	Noncarbonated filtered water with fresh lemon or lime
Ice cream	Frozen organic soy dessert (no sugar added)

Chapter Summary

Eating healthful nutritious foods need not be any more expensive or inconvenient than consuming processed prepackaged foods. You simply need to organize your kitchen and learn a few basic techniques. Your reward for commitment can be a lifetime of feeling vibrant and disease free; as Hippocrates so judiciously surmised, food is medicine.

Half the nutrition battle is keeping the right foods and cooking tools stocked and ready for immediate and convenient use, while banning the wrong foods from your kitchen entirely. The ten recommendations described in this chapter give you all the information you will need about what to do and how to do it.

Ten Practical Ways to Perform a Healthy Kitchen Makeover

1. Invest in quality tools to make cooking easier. Organize your kitchen to make accessing these tools convenient.

2. Inventory your pantry, refrigerator, freezer, and cupboards, and donate (or eliminate) any unhealthy foods you find lurking in your house or apartment.

3. Replace the processed foods you disposed of during your kitchen makeover with fresh whole foods.

4. Plan your menus weekly to maximize variety and vitality in your diet. Make sure to complete your weekly menu plan before you go out to shop for food.

5. When cooking, make extra of each item for leftovers to use throughout the rest of the week.

6. Make cooking fun and social—invite a friend to cook with you, or make cooking a family event and include lots of fun for the kids.

7. Do not feel obliged to make everything from scratch. Use quality prepared food items when necessary.

8. Listen to soothing music or watch a relaxing TV show as "background" if cooking alone. Do not watch anything distressing or distracting.

9. Create or try a new recipe each week to keep a little spice in your life.

10. Rewrite all your favorite unhealthy recipes. You can transform each one into a much more healthful recipe by substituting selected ingredients.

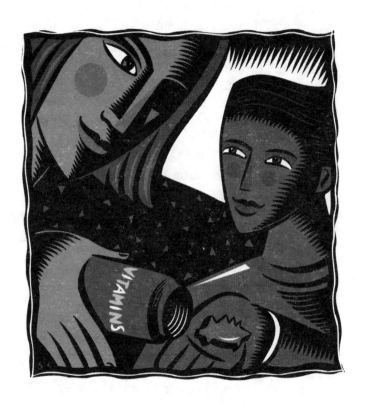

For optimum nutrition, supplementation is a necessity for all people—regardless of age, race, or gender.

Key Factor Six
Supplement Your Diet with
Quality Vitamins and Minerals

I was taught to believe that I could receive all the vitamins and minerals I needed to stay healthy from the foods I ate. If you read my introduction to the chapter on nutritious meals, you know that the foods I used to eat were far from being nutrient rich. But, just to cover my bases, I would purchase the least expensive multivitamin from the drugstore (and later, from the discount warehouse).

It wasn't until I learned about the differences between a pharmaceutical-grade supplement and the commercial brands that I was convinced I wasn't getting the full benefits from my inadequate supplementation program. I researched doctors who knew about quality vitamins, minerals, and herbs who had patients they helped through a complete supplementation program. I began taking a recommended brand that was based on science and quality, not on mass commercialization, and I saw and felt the difference within a few months.

I have made supplementation part of my daily routine. After witnessing my recovery from lupus and fibromyalgia, my husband and other family members have made taking quality supplements a part of their lives as well.

Even if you don't think you are at risk for any health issues, and even if you feel perfectly healthy today, quality supplements can help you maintain your health and enhance your immunity.

—*Jodi L. Jones*

In recent years, the tide has turned in the traditional medical community toward supporting the benefits of vitamin and mineral supplements.[1,2] While the research is clear, the quality of nutritional supplements in the United States varies greatly. In Europe, government controls supplements in the same way as prescription drugs, but in this country we have the benefits of easily available, inexpensive supplements. The lack of oversight and regulation in the United States has produced poor reliability about what is stated on the label and raises the question, "Is the contents of the bottle delivering all that it claims?"

Although there are a number of excellent brands of nutritional supplements, in my opinion, there are many poor brands. I have recommended just a few specific brands in Appendix C to help you create an effective vitality program.

—*Michael J. Grossman, M.D.*

Many people ask the question, "If I eat balanced, nutritious meals every day, do I need to take supplements? Can't I get the nutrients I need from food?" The short answer is "no."[3-5] Well, technically, it is possible to get complete nutrient value from foods. However, you would have to eat such an exorbitant amount of the right types of foods, it would not physically be possible. For example, the following table compares the amount of each food item you would have to consume to receive an optimal daily amount of vitamin E, one of the most powerful antioxidants:

Food	To Obtain 400 IU
Sunflower seeds	1.2 lbs.
Wheat germ	5.2 lbs.
Almonds	2.2 lbs.
Safflower oil	1 quart
Spinach	33 Lbs.

Due to modern agricultural practices that have been driven to value profit much more highly than nutrition, our croplands have been depleted of essential minerals and micronutrients. The nutritional value of cultivated foods is at an all-time low. To compound this issue of subnutrition prevalent in whole foods and grains, the majority of nonwhole foods consumed today are processed, packaged, and loaded with carcinogenic chemicals, preservatives, and dyes. Processed foods and commercially prepared meals are simply devoid of adequate nutritional value.[6] The increase in toxic heavy metals, industrial pollutants, chemical waste, and environmental toxins also contributes to the need for supplementation.[7]

As discussed in Key Factor One on anti-aging, your body is attacked by more than 100,000 hits of free radicals daily from external and internal sources. These damaged molecules injure your cell walls, DNA, enzymes, and mitochondria. Left unchecked, these free radicals can cause chain reactions and explosions that create massive damage and shift the aging process into high gear. To protect your body, you must consume food and nutritional supplements containing high levels of antioxidants that bind to and neutralize free radicals at the molecular level, rendering them relatively harmless.

Scientific research indicates that to attain optimum nutrition for good health and vitality, people of all ages must supplement their diets with quality vitamins, minerals, and herbs. The relationship between nutrition and health has long been recognized.

Before 1960, interest in this field was primarily focused on the benefits of nutrients to prevent diseases such as scurvy and rickets. As a result of this research, fifty essential nutrients such as vitamins, minerals, antioxidants, cofactors, essential amino acids, and essential fatty acids, were identified and Recommended Dietary Allowances (RDAs) were established.

Research has proliferated over the past few decades and more and more clinical studies have been centered on the impact of nutrition on chronic degenerative diseases such as heart disease, arthritis, and Type 2 diabetes, as well as some cancers and autoimmune disorders. [8-11]

Based on scientific findings, we know that supplements deliver a wealth of health benefits if taken at an optimum level of five to ten times the RDA levels previously mentioned. Supplementation, together with proper diet and exercise, has been shown to:

- Protect DNA.
- Neutralize free-radical damage.
- Enhance mental function.

- Aid in the prevention of cancer.
- Reduce the risk of cardiovascular and other diseases.
- Improve emotional disorders.
- Enhance immune function.
- Strengthen nails.
- Improve skin elasticity.

Supplements may be beneficial in improving the efficiency of just about every system in your body. It is important to note that mainstream medical doctors, for the most part, are not trained or educated on the benefits of supplementation. More and more doctors, however, are realizing the number of health benefits attained from the consumption of quality nutritional supplementation.

To attain the full benefits, you must consume quality supplements that are not only balanced in nutrient values but are also readily absorbed by the body. Also, to get the most out of your supplementation program, it is critical to take certain vitamins and minerals together and in the right proportions. Many vitamins and minerals require the presence of other nutrients, known as cofactors, in order to work effectively.

Appendix C contains a chart containing recommended dosages for dozens of vitamin, mineral, and herbal supplements. The same chart lists cofactors that should be present for maximum absorption of each nutrient. Use this section at the back of the book as a reference tool when putting together your own supplementation regimen. Appendix C also lists recommended brands from reputable science-based supplement manufacturers who have developed quality supplements in balanced proportions, taking the guesswork out for you.

Ten Practical Ways to Supplement Your Diet

1. Purchase only the highest quality bioavailable supplements that guarantee potency and meet GMP and USP standards.

You might be asking yourself, "What is bioavailability and why is it important?" One good definition of bioavailability is the amount of a nutrient ingested that is absorbed and therefore available to the body for metabolic use. Bioavailability is important because all nutritional intake must be available to various body systems for growth, maintenance of body tissues, reproduction, and other performance factors. No matter how high the nutrient levels or how well formulated the product, if it is not bioavailable, money and effort have been wasted.

Many commercial brands of supplements on supermarket and drugstore shelves do not meet the quality standards, potency, safety, and proper nutrient balance needed to provide even minimal health benefits. How efficiently and effectively a supplement dissolves and is absorbed is critical. Lower quality supplements can pass through the digestive system only partially absorbed or still intact.

High-quality supplements are formulated to effectively balance the minerals present so trace minerals can be absorbed. Additionally, high-quality supplements provide a balanced ratio of vitamins and minerals needed for optimum health and are guaranteed for potency, safety, and uniformity. This means each and every tablet or capsule is equally potent and safe.

There are many factors to consider when selecting a quality nutritional supplement. Just as important as the particular brand of supplement is the reliability and reputation of the manufacturer. The following are six very important questions to ask of the vitamin manufacturer:

1. Are the supplements scientifically formulated and balanced with the proper ratio of nutrients?

2. Do they follow Good Manufacturing Practices (GMP) and comply with U.S. Pharmacological (USP) Standards for pharmaceutical-grade products? *Since the FDA does not regulate potency or safety of supplements, it is important to consume brands that meet USP and GMP Standards.*

3. Are they independently tested and guaranteed for potency and safety? *This is an important question because what you read on the label does not guarantee what is in the product.*

4. Are they manufactured in-house by a reputable company with ongoing scientific research and development? *This is important because many companies contract to an outside generic supplement manufacturer, usually the lowest bidder, and simply put their label on the bottle.*

5. Is the product recommended by nutrition-oriented medical doctors?

6. Are the nutrients provided in their most bioavailable and therefore most absorbable form?

2. Take your supplements with food and water to ensure optimum absorption. Reference the water-soluble versus fat-soluble table.

For maximum absorption of most minerals and vitamins, take your supplements with food. The presence of food in your stomach releases acids that increase nutrient absorption; fats and oils present in your food will transport fat-soluble vitamins. Water is also a factor in absorption and can limit the impact that high-dose vitamin and mineral supplements cause on the digestive system. If you experience digestive upsets or bloating when you take supplements, increase the amount of water you drink and see if this problem goes away.

The following table provides a general overview of which vitamins and minerals are best absorbed with water (water soluble) versus foods (fat soluble):

Water-Soluble Nutrients

Vitamin B_1

Vitamin B_2

Vitamin B_3

Vitamin B_5

Vitamin B_6

Vitamin B_{12}

Vitamin C

Folic Acid

Biotin

Fat-Soluble Nutrients

Vitamin A

Vitamin E

Vitamin D

Coenzyme Q10

3. Consume supplements in small amounts throughout the day, or as directed.

Read the label on your supplement bottle and take as directed. If you ingest all your vitamins and minerals at one sitting, you will be severely taxing your intestines' ability to absorb so many minerals and vitamins at one time. In addition, some minerals compete with each other for absorption. When you take all your minerals at once, you will absorb the dominant higher dose minerals, such as calcium and magnesium, but will be unable to absorb trace minerals, such as selenium.

4. Consult with a health practitioner regarding possible drug interactions.

Some vitamins, minerals, and herbs can accentuate or impede the effectiveness of prescription drugs. If you are currently taking prescription drugs, it is essential to consult with a medical professional so that you are aware of all potential drug interactions. Schedule this consultation before you begin a rigorous supplementation regimen.

Aspirin, birth control pills, hormone replacement therapy, and antibiotics can all increase the need for certain supplements, such as beneficial bacteria, vitamin C, and B vitamins; check with your physician for dosage recommendations.

If you are currently taking blood thinners, you should refrain from taking fish oil, vitamin E, vitamin K, ginkgo biloba, glucosamine/chondroitin sulfate, and virtually all herbs unless physician advised, as they too can cause further thinning of the blood. Anticonvulsants can increase your need for folic acid. St. John's wort may speed the elimination of many prescription drugs, making the drugs less effective.

This list of potential adverse reactions is just a sampling of possible drug interactions when combining supplements with prescription drugs. Avoid negative side effects and do not risk reducing the effectiveness of expensive prescription medications. Schedule a consultation with a health practitioner *before* you begin your supplementation regimen.

5. If you are taking supplements to build bone density, measure the effectiveness of your program by means of medical testing.

Women should begin monitoring their bodies for signs of osteoporosis by regular bone density testing, establishing baseline results for comparison purposes, at thirty-five years of age. It is also recommended that women over age forty be tested yearly. Contrary to what many may think, men are certainly not immune to osteoporosis and would benefit by being tested annually after fifty-five years of age.

The standard for osteoporosis testing is the Dexa X-ray of the spine and hip that gives a small amount of X-ray exposure. An option that avoids radiation is the heel ultrasound testing, which is extremely accurate when it comes to measuring the small changes that occur from one year to the next. These changes are the most critical aspect of bone density testing to determine if you are losing bone mass.

If testing reveals loss of bone density, there are several things you can do to reverse the trend. Calcium is an excellent supplement to take. Exercise is also a necessary activity as it not only builds muscle mass, but also builds bone density. Bear in mind that weight lifting is more critical to building bone density than aerobic exercise. Refer to the chapter on exercise for more details.

6. Supplement your diet with vitamins A, C, and E, the three most critical antioxidants.

The cells of your body are under daily attack by a strike force of upwards of 100,000 free radicals every day from pollution, smoke, radiation, fried foods, exhaust fumes, and normal body processes. If you do not mount an effective defense against free radicals, your chances of contracting a host of degenerative diseases are greatly increased. Antioxidants play a critical part in maintaining physiological health and reducing the effects of aging by neutralizing this onslaught of free radicals.

The three primary antioxidants are vitamins A, C, and E. Vitamin A not only boosts the immune system and protects against infections, but it is also effective at cancer prevention. Vitamin A is also beneficial for night vision and healthy skin.

Vitamin A can be toxic in large amounts; pregnant women should not take more than 5,000 units daily, and children under age four should consume fewer than 2,500 units per day. Additionally, it is important to note that this only applies to preformed vitamin A. Carotenoids are considered to be safe and nontoxic at almost any dose. They may turn you orange, doubly so for individuals with thyroid disease, but remain safe. This is confusing because current labeling laws require manufacturers to list the vitamin A activity of beta-carotene in their products, when in truth, the body will stop converting when tissue levels of vitamin A are saturated.

Substances known as carotenoids are found in numerous fruits and vegetables; these are converted by the body into active vitamin A (primarily beta-carotene). Carrots, one of the best food sources of vitamin A, contain more than twenty different carotenoids. Beta-carotene is only one of these carotenoids; since it is relatively inexpensive, beta-carotene is most commonly found in multivitamin supplements. When shopping for a multivitamin, for best effectiveness look for mixed carotenoids, not just beta-carotene.[12]

Vitamin C aids in the body's production of collagen, for strong joints, bones, and skin. Vitamin C has been shown to prevent cancer and heart disease and helps the body manufacture anti stress hormones. For vitamin C to function to its full capacity, take it with its bioflavonoid cofactor. Sources include citrus fruits, pine tree bark, and grapeseed extract; top-quality multivitamins will include bioflavonoids to maximize the power of vitamin C. It is worth noting that many of the bioflavonoids are powerful antioxidants in their own right.

Vitamin E promotes healthy skin and rapid healing of wounds. Vitamin E also protects cells from injury, including cancer. By helping the body utilize oxygen more effectively, vitamin E also guards against atherosclerosis, thrombosis, and blood clots. Check the label on your multivitamin bottle to see if your supplements contain natural vitamin E as d-alpha-tocopherol or synthetic vitamin E as dl-alpha. The synthetic form is less active and less effective. Also, when taking more than 200 units of vitamin E, it is best to take a mix of gamma and delta as well as alpha-tocopherol.

7. Supplement your diet with other essential vitamins: vitamins D, K, and B complex.

The B vitamins include B_1 (thiamine), B_2 (riboflavin), B_3 (niacin), B_5 (pantothenic acid), B_6 (pyridoxine), and B_{12} (cyanocobalamin). In addition to these B vitamins, B complex typically includes biotin and folic acid, also essential nutrients. The B vitamins have a wide range of functions in the body including oxygen transport, protein utilization, improved brain function, energy production, and maintenance of healthy skin and nails, to name only a few. Clearly, a daily dose of B complex is a vital part of any supplementation regimen. Do not take B complex, however, at bedtime, since it promotes energy and may keep you awake.

Vitamin D is vital for its role in retaining calcium and keeping bones healthy and strong. Since the skin manufactures vitamin D when it is exposed to sunlight, supplementation of this vitamin may not be necessary if you spend a lot of time outdoors. It is important to be cautious about exposing your skin to excessive levels of ultraviolet rays. Too much direct exposure can increase your risk for skin cancer and other health problems. To minimize damage, be sure to apply sunscreen with a minimum of SPF 30 every few hours to exposed areas of the skin.

Vitamin K helps the body synthesize proteins necessary for blood clotting. It has recently been shown to help keep bones strong and help prevent arteriosclerosis and heart disease. Vitamin K may be a relative unknown among vitamins and highly specialized in its benefits, yet it still has earned its place in the essential vitamin category.

8. Supplement your diet with the essential minerals, calcium and magnesium.

When it comes to the benefits it can deliver, calcium goes beyond building strong teeth and bones. Calcium also plays an important role in heart health and nerve function and may be helpful in reducing menstrual cramps.

Not all forms of calcium are created equal, and there are several forms from which to choose. All forms of calcium can reduce bone loss, but the only form of calcium that has been shown to actually build bone density is called Cal-Apatite, or microcrystalline hydroxyapatite; this form is produced by grinding up frozen cow bones and maintaining the protein matrix attached to the calcium. When it comes to absorption, calcium glycinate is the next most bioavailable form, followed by calcium citrate.

Even though you need between 1,000 and 1,500 mg daily, human intestines can only absorb 600 mg of calcium at one time. Spread your dose throughout the day to ensure that you are absorbing all the calcium you need.

Magnesium must be available for building bone and is a necessary component for heart and nervous system health. Most adults are deficient in magnesium. One common mistake people make is to take calcium without magnesium.

Take half as much magnesium as you take of calcium to ensure proper absorption. It is actually best to buy a quality calcium supplement that includes the proper balance of magnesium already in the tablet. Also, when purchasing calcium and magnesium supplements, look for chelated forms. Both calcium and magnesium are best absorbed as chelated glycinate.

Taking the bulk of your mineral supplements at bedtime can have a beneficial side effect. Minerals are better absorbed while you sleep; they also have a relaxing effect on the muscles that can help you rest better.

9. Supplement your diet with trace minerals: zinc, iron, copper, manganese, boron, chromium, selenium, iodine, silicon, and vanadium.

The problem with absorption of trace minerals is competition. Large doses of calcium and magnesium can overwhelm the body's ability to absorb the other minerals. Look for chelated minerals when choosing supplements containing iron, zinc, copper, manganese, magnesium, calcium, and chromium. Chelated minerals offer much improved absorption rates.[13,14] When these minerals become surrounded by and bonded to amino acids, in a stable form, this is called chelation. Chelation is a natural means for the body to transport minerals across the intestinal wall as part of digestion. Refer to Appendix C for recommended brands based on scientific studies.

The following list describes the various trace minerals and reasons why they are important:

- **Zinc.** Zinc protects and maintains DNA, assists in the healing process, helps balance hormones, and increases energy levels.
- **Iron.** Iron is essential in energy production and oxygen transport. Deficiency can cause fatigue. Too much iron can rob you of zinc.

- **Copper.** Copper is necessary in the formation of nerve sheaths; deficiency of this mineral has been linked to rheumatoid arthritis. An excess of copper consumption is toxic so you need to be cautious in supplementation; you may be getting more than enough copper from the copper plumbing in your home.
- **Manganese.** Manganese is needed for the proper functioning of the brain and more than twenty enzyme systems in the body. It may also promote joint health.
- **Boron.** Boron may help maintain healthy calcium balance, possibly through involvement in estrogen and vitamin D metabolism. It may also promote brain health as well.
- **Chromium.** Chromium helps establish healthy glucose metabolism, balances blood sugar, and promotes a healthy heart and DNA.
- **Selenium.** When you take into account selenium's effectiveness in fighting carcinogens and free radicals, the single most effective thing you can do to aid in the prevention of cancer is to take 200 mcg of this trace mineral daily. For this small cost there is roughly a 50 percent reduction in the incidence of cancer.
- **Iodine.** Iodine is required for healthy thyroid function. Iodine is a common ingredient in multivitamin supplements; however, you can also get your iodine needs met by using iodized salt on your food.
- **Silicon.** Silicon may be important for healthy bones and for making and maintaining connective tissue.
- **Vanadium.** Researchers believe that vanadium may improve cholesterol levels and help people with insulin resistance transport glucose into the cells.

10. Supplement your diet with the key semi essential nutrients: coenzyme Q10, bioflavonoids, and fish oil.

- **Coenzyme Q10 (CoQ10).** CoQ10 is a powerful antioxidant and has a key role in aiding the body to metabolize energy. Cardiovascular benefits include improved heart function, regulation of blood pressure, and boosted exercise tolerance. As we get into our forties, we lose the ability to produce CoQ10 in sufficient amounts.
- **Bioflavonoids.** The presence of bioflavonoids increases the body's absorption of vitamin C. In addition to their antioxidant properties, bioflavonoids can help strengthen capillaries and promote rapid healing.
- **Omega-3 oils** from fish may be the single best nutrient for longer life as they have been shown to reduce heart disease and decrease clotting tendency.
- **Concentrated nutrients** from broccoli, tomato, garlic, turmeric, and ginger have a number of health benefits. Many products have concentrates that may prevent heart disease, cancer, and arthritis.

Refer to Appendix C for information on dosages, cofactors, and dietary sources of vitamins, minerals, and omega-3 oils.

Chapter Summary

The nutritional value of cultivated foods is at an all-time low, and the consumption of processed and fast foods is at an all-time high. It is just not possible to receive adequate nutrient value from the foods you eat. In order to optimize health and vitality, everyone needs to take quality vitamin, mineral, and herbal supplements to make their diets complete.

Supplements have been shown to protect DNA, improve mental acuity, enhance digestion, and aid in the prevention of cancer and many degenerative diseases, among many other health benefits.

To achieve noticeable and lasting results, you must take quality supplements that are manufactured by a company that guarantees potency, bioavailability, and safety. It is also important to use products that provide the proper balance and optimum ratio of vitamins and minerals. At a minimum, take balanced multivitamins and chelated minerals each day.

There are few commercial retail brands of nutritional supplements that meet the quality standards, potency, and proper nutrient ratios required to protect your cells.[15-17] Therefore, for optimum benefit, consult a nutrition-focused health practitioner or trained nutritional consultant for recommendations on quality supplements.

There are numerous factors to consider before engaging in an effective supplementation regimen. The ten recommendations below provide highlights of what you need to know.

Ten Practical Ways to Supplement Your Diet

1. Purchase only the highest quality bioavailable supplements that guarantee potency and meet GMP and USP Standards.
2. Take your supplements with food and water to ensure optimum absorption. Reference the water-soluble versus fat-soluble table.

3. Consume supplements in small amounts throughout the day, or as directed.
4. Consult with a health practitioner regarding possible drug interactions.
5. If you are taking supplements to build bone density, measure the effectiveness of your program by means of medical testing.
6. Supplement your diet with vitamins A, C, and E, the three most critical antioxidants.
7. Supplement your diet with other essential vitamins: vitamins D, K, and B complex.
8. Supplement your diet with the essential minerals: calcium and magnesium.
9. Supplement your diet with trace minerals: zinc, iron, copper, manganese, boron, chromium, selenium, iodine, silicon, and vanadium.
10. Supplement your diet with key semi essential nutrients: coenzyme Q10, bioflavonoids, and fish oil.

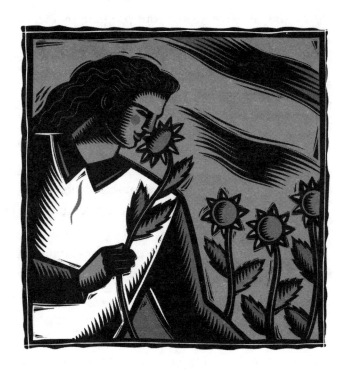

Immune system balance is a key to unlocking many of the mysteries of chronic illness—the key is within your reach.

Key Factor Seven
Balance Your Immune System

As a physician in 1980, I laughed when I first heard that overgrowth of yeast in the gastrointestinal tract could be a cause of chronic illness. I remember thinking; every physician knows that yeast is a harmless organism.

Some years later I learned that, in some individuals, yeast can irritate and aggravate the immune system and the gastrointestinal lining and thereby create serious illness. It was very humbling to find myself in the camp of those whose theories I once found ludicrous.

Most medical doctors today are still ignorant about the gastrointestinal tract's role in balancing the immune system. As an assistant clinical professor at the medical school of the University of California at Irvine, however, I lecture and teach medical students, interns, and residents. These young and upcoming physicians are extremely interested in the body of knowledge presented in these chapters.

I assure you, I have employed these methods a thousand times with chronically ill patients with consistent and repeatable improvements.

—Michael J. Grossman, M.D.

Immune System Assessment

To determine your immune system balance, answer each of the following questions in Part 1 and Part 2 with a "yes" or "no."

PART I

Do you have any of the following symptoms?

Joint pains

Muscle aches

Gastrointestinal upsets—stomach pain after eating

Diarrhea

Constipation—bowels do not move every day, or stools are hard and dry

Gas and bloating

Poor digestion—food repeats on you after eating (belching)

Poor appetite

Bad odor from stool

Mood swings

Headaches—more than once a month

Catch colds easily

Skin rashes—your skin itches often

Asthma

Chronic cough

Sinus congestion—a need to clear your throat often

Any "yes" answer in Part I suggests you need to read and apply the recommendations in this chapter.

PART II

Do you:

Eat high-fiber foods several times daily?

Ingest good bacteria such as lactobacillus acidophilus and bifida bacteria?

Eat fresh whole foods, such as fruits, vegetables, legumes, and beans
several times daily?

Ingest a quality source of omega-3 oils daily?

Sleep enough daily?

*Any "no" answer in Part II suggests you need to read and apply the rec-
ommendations in this chapter.*

Your body is not a closed, sealed system. In the course of
eating, drinking, and breathing, you come into contact with a
world full of bacteria, fungi, viruses, dirt, dust, pesticides,
foods and food contaminants, pollutants, pollen, and toxins.
To survive and continue functioning normally, your body must
neutralize foreign substances and organisms.

Manufacturing and distributing antibodies to ward off disease is the job of your immune system. The lymph tissue is the
mechanism by which the body stores immune information
regarding every foreign substance the immune system has
ever encountered. As substances enter, the memory banks are
searched so that the immune system can manufacture and dispatch the right antibody to kill them.

The Intestinal Tract: Key to Balancing the Immune System

Although some substances and organisms enter your body
through the nose and respiratory tract, most enter through the
mouth, the gateway to the intestines. So it is not surprising that
60 to 70 percent of your lymph tissue is located around the
intestinal tract.

Although you cannot easily control everything you breathe
in, you can control what you eat. Balancing the immune system is possible by controlling what you eat in order to create

a healthy gastrointestinal tract and healthy gastrointestinal bacterial flora.

Your small intestines are about twenty-seven feet long and only about three inches in diameter. When you take into account fingerlike projections called villi, however, the total surface area of your gastrointestinal tract is larger than a tennis court.

Prolonged imbalance of the immune system leads to inflammation throughout the body, a major contributor to accelerated aging and life-threatening autoimmune disorders. If your immune system is overfunctioning, it promotes autoimmune diseases. If your immune system is underfunctioning, it leaves you susceptible to infections. That is why restoring proper balance is so critical.

At the far extreme of immune system imbalance are people who have been diagnosed with autoimmune disorders such as lupus, rheumatoid arthritis, ulcerative colitis, and thyroiditis. The immune systems of autoimmune disease sufferers may become so out of balance that they produce antibodies and dispatch them to attack their own internal organs.

A major cause of immune system imbalance is leaky gut syndrome.[1-4] Chronic gastrointestinal inflammation can cause increased permeability of the intestinal lining. When the "cement" between cells in the lining of the intestines becomes loosened, particles that would normally be eliminated are able to pass right through the intestinal wall and directly into the bloodstream. When the gut becomes leaky, the body is forced to make repeated attempts to process and neutralize the same contaminants and toxins, creating high amounts of stress within your body.

When your diet is low in fiber and high in sugar, your immune system can be imbalanced due to overgrowth of yeast and unhealthy bacteria. The by-products of yeast metabolism and unhealthy bacteria can cause inflammation in the gastrointestinal tract and throughout the body. [5]

Creating a healthy gastrointestinal tract requires four stages, says advanced nutrition researcher Dr. Jeffrey Bland: remove, replace, repopulate, and repair. Dr. Bland has defined the protocols for treatment to include: [6]

- Remove harmful bacteria, yeast, and parasites.
- Replace digestive enzymes and/or hydrochloric acid.
- Repopulate the healthy gastrointestinal bacteria.
- Repair the cells of the injured intestinal lining.

Repairing the intestinal lining is a gradual process that incorporates the ten recommendations that follow.

Ten Practical Ways to Balance Your Immune System

1. To improve your digestion, treat abdominal gas and bloating with digestive enzymes and other digestive aids.

There is a grain of truth to the saying, "You are what you eat." In the interest of accuracy, however, the statement needs to be expanded to, "You are what you are able to digest and absorb." In addition, you must suffer the consequences of whatever you ingest but are not able to properly digest and absorb.

Improper or incomplete digestion not only contributes to imbalance of the immune system, but also to a host of other adverse effects:

- Decreased absorption of nutrients
- Inefficient elimination of toxins and wastes
- Elevated concentrations of toxins and contaminants
- Inflammation of the intestinal tract
- Impaired organ function and organ system stress
- Compromised utilization of oxygen and production of energy
- Degeneration of tissue and cells

Some people have difficulty digesting specific types of foods, such as milk, beans, protein, or fat. Enzymes, chemical compounds that break down large food particles into smaller units, are essential to the process of digesting and absorbing what you eat. If you are lactose-intolerant, for example, you may need to take the enzyme lactase before eating dairy products and milk in order to adequately break down the milk sugar lactose.

The following supplements may aid you in digesting certain foods:

- Pepsin, betaine hydrochloride, protease, and the herb gentian can improve digestion of protein.
- Amylase and other enzymes can help you better digest starches.
- Lipase and bile salts can improve digestion of fats.
- Beano is an enzyme helpful for digesting beans.
- Gentian is an herb that aids acid production and improves digestion in general.

You will know the enzymes are working when you no longer experience gas and bloating. Start out with low dosages and gradually increase them until you obtain some relief.

Sometimes digestive difficulties are caused by low stomach acid. Many people feel pain after they eat because they have too little acid, not too much. As people get older, they lose the ability to produce acid: over 50 percent of people aged sixty-five and older have too little acid and can benefit from supplementation.

Ironically, most people suffering from indigestion will run to the pharmacy and self-administer an acid neutralizer, such as Rolaids or Tums, which may only aggravate the condition. When indigestion strikes, what you may need is a hydrochloric acid supplement, in the form of betaine HCl. As a last resort, if there are certain foods you absolutely cannot eat without experiencing acute gas and bloating, you should eliminate those foods from your diet.

2. Restore good bacteria in your intestinal tract by taking capsules containing vibrant good bacteria.

There are trillions of bacteria in your gastrointestinal tract; that is more bacteria than cells in your body, or stars in the known universe. Taking vibrant good bacteria, both lactobacillus acidophilus and bifida bacteria in capsule form, is key to restoring good bacteria in your intestinal tract.[7,8] It is important to note that these organisms are alive and that they must stay that way; the capsules require refrigeration.

Good bacteria are essential for intestinal health. They help your body produce vitamin K and B vitamins. Their metabolism creates by-products, butyrate and L-glutamine, that nourish the lining of the intestinal tract. Balanced bacterial flora keep your gut healthy and improve digestion and elimination. When bacteria are imbalanced, by-products are created that irritate the lining of the intestinal tract. This irritation can cause diarrhea, leaky gut syndrome, immune imbalance, oxidative stress, liver toxicity, and chronic fatigue. Diarrhea promotes ill health by causing food to pass through your system too quickly before the nutrients can be absorbed.

In your supermarket's dairy case, you may have noticed milk and yogurt containing acidophilus, which is not useful for the purposes described here. Commercial yogurt contains bacteria that taste good but are not vibrant, hardy bacteria that will grow in your gastrointestinal tract. A serving of acidophilus milk or yogurt contains hundreds of thousands of good bacteria; to receive the real benefits of good bacteria, you need billions. You can only obtain this quantity from the concentrated capsule form. When purchasing capsules, look for the NCFM strain of acidophilus (discovered in North Carolina's Food Microbiology unit), which research has shown to grow successfully in the human gastrointestinal tract.

It is especially important to ingest good bacteria for a month after taking antibiotics, as this form of treatment kills both the good and bad bacteria in your system. You need to replenish the good bacteria destroyed by the antibiotics.

3. Eat foods that are high in insoluble fiber to prevent constipation and eliminate toxins from the intestinal tract.

There are two types of fiber: soluble and insoluble. Insoluble fiber (for example, wheat bran and the cellulose content present in grains and vegetables) passes through your intestinal tract intact without being digested. Insoluble fiber acts like a broom brushing the inside of your intestines clean and potentially sweeping out toxins, contaminants, and undigested and putrefied food. Insoluble fiber can be your best defense against constipation. Having two to four large bowel movements per day is an important way to keep the body from accumulating toxins.

4. Ingest enough soluble fiber to nourish your intestinal lining and feed good bacteria.

If you withhold soluble fiber from your good bacteria, your intestinal tract can starve. This kind of damage to your intestinal lining is the first step to developing leaky gut syndrome.

Soluble fiber is necessary for good bacteria to produce butyrate and L-glutamine, which your intestinal lining needs for nourishment. When you ingest high levels of both soluble and insoluble fiber, you can reduce your risk for many diseases, such as diverticulitis, colitis, and colon cancer. Good sources of soluble fiber include whole grains, beans, fresh vegetables and fruits, and raw nuts and seeds. Inulin fiber from Jerusalem artichokes is particularly helpful in stimulating the growth of good bacteria and the production of fuel for the intestinal lining.

5. Eliminate yeast, parasites, and harmful bacteria by eating less sugar and taking specific herbs.

Many people are extremely sensitive to yeast, *Candida*, and yeast by-products, which can cause irritation and injury to the intestinal tract and the entire body.

Bacteria and yeast compete with each other for food. Each secretes substances toxic to the other, with the objective of killing off its rival and gaining full control of food sources.

Mitochondria, the power packs present by the thousands inside all of our cells, are very easily injured by the by-products of yeast metabolism. Mitochondria are not easily repaired. When such injury impairs mitochondrial function, the result can be extreme fatigue.

Eliminating refined sugar, their food source, can control yeast. In addition, the presence of good bacteria and fiber will gradually crowd out yeast and other imbalancing organisms. A variety of herbs and prescription medicines may also be required to eliminate irritating and unhealthy amounts of bacteria. Recommended herbs include uva ursi and grapefruit seed extract, berberine, oregano leaf extract, and red thyme oil.

Minor parasites (such as *Bastocystis hominis*) can irritate and inflame the gastrointestinal tract. While herbs can help, prescription medicines may be necessary in some cases. Work with health professionals and consider taking a stool specimen for evaluation of imbalanced bacteria, yeast, and parasites. See Appendix B for laboratories that do a comprehensive stool evaluation.

6. Eat whole natural foods that are very fresh; the fresher the food, the more the enzymes in the food can help you with nutrient digestion and absorption.

The enzymes that are present in all whole foods, which can be a great aid to digestion, become less effective with age. This fact underscores the dietary need for fresh organic whole foods, as opposed to heat-processed, refined, and preserved foods.

If fruits and vegetables have been sitting on your kitchen counter or refrigerator shelf for weeks, they are not optimally contributing to improved digestion. A healthy habit to develop is to go to the market more frequently, instead of buying large quantities of whole fresh food items that will take a week or more to consume.

7. Improve gastrointestinal health with L-glutamine.

If you have problems with gastrointestinal symptoms, you may need to restore the lining of the GI tract to full vibrant thickness to aid in absorption and to repair leaky gut syndrome. The amino acid L-glutamine is the necessary food for the lining of the small intestines. Doses range from 500 mg three times daily to 3,000 mg four times daily.

Other nutrients can help repair an irritated or leaky GI tract including zinc, N-acetylcysteine, and other antioxidants, such as selenium and vitamins A, C, and E. For a listing of recommended products, see Appendix C.

8. Follow a rotation or elimination diet to keep food allergies from causing gastrointestinal irritation and immune imbalance.

Food allergies are a very common cause of irritation to the gastrointestinal tract.[9] Generally speaking, if there is a type of food that you crave and absolutely must have on a daily basis, the chances are good that you are allergic to it. [10–12]

Foods that you are allergic to can be great irritants to the intestinal tract and typically can cause problems with inflammation, injury to mitochondria and cells, and excess immune activation. In addition, food allergies may cause fatigue, mood swings, muscle and joint pain, headaches, respiratory conditions, rashes, asthma, and abdominal pain. If you have recurrent problems in any of these areas, you may benefit greatly from an elimination or rotation diet.

Many of the allergic symptoms listed above are quite noticeable; however, they may exhibit a delayed reaction, appearing up to several days after the food has been eaten. The elimination diet followed by the rotation diet helps pinpoint specific foods as causes of allergic reactions.

In an elimination diet, you eliminate specific allergens, such as dairy, wheat and other grains, or beef, for a period of at least five days before rotating in previously eliminated foods. It takes about four days for an allergen to work out of your system and for withdrawal from that food to be complete. If you notice withdrawal symptoms (such as headaches or muscle and joint pains) during the first four days, and then feel really great on day five, you have probably identified a food allergy.

The primary benefit of an elimination diet is to clear your body of toxins. Many people are sensitive to dairy and wheat; the elimination diet calls for complete avoidance of dairy products. You also eliminate gluten, by avoiding any food containing wheat or other grains and flours including oats, barley, rye, amaranth, spelt, kamut, quinoa, or malts.

On an elimination diet, you also avoid eating red meat and foods containing yeast or foods that promote yeast overgrowth. Foods promoting overgrowth of yeast include sugar, processed foods, and most foods that come in a box or bottle. The last tenet of an elimination diet concerns healthy beverage choices. Eliminate alcoholic beverages and any beverages containing caffeine; be sure to drink at least two quarts of water daily.

Follow this elimination diet for eight to twenty-one days. While you are eliminating many foods completely, you are allowed to eat fish and fowl, healthy fats, fruits, and vegetables. For grains, you can choose rice, millet, or buckwheat. Your health practitioner may advocate the use of a medical fiber beverage that can aid detoxification without further inflaming your intestines. At the end of eight to twenty-one days, your system will be at least partially cleared of toxic substances and you may feel better than you have in years.

At the end of the elimination diet, you can begin rotating the previously banned foods back into your diet to observe their effects on your body. Some people can eat previously allergy-causing foods once every week and not have any significant reactions. For these people, eating the food two times a week is more likely to cause an allergic reaction to develop. Other people have an immediate reaction anytime they eat the offending food. This process can indicate your individual food sensitivities and allergies. Use the results of these food experiments to create an optimal diet for your individual metabolism—one that can free you permanently from the harmful effects of food sensitivities and allergies.

9. Reduce inflammation by eliminating bad fats from your diet and increasing your intake of healthy fats.

While the optimal intake of fat in the diet is 20 to 30 percent of total calories, the average person ingests up to 40 percent. This level is far too high to support optimal health. If you are at this average level or above and are consuming red meat, dairy products including butter, and fried foods, you are getting too much unhealthy fat.

The figure below presents fat sources ranked by their positive and negative effects. At the top is the best source for reducing inflammation, fish oil. At the bottom you will find the worst fat sources for causing inflammation: refined oils, margarine, and trans fats.

Fats That Reduce Inflammation

Fish oil

Hemp

Flax

Soybeans

Walnuts

Sunflower seeds

Almonds

Evening primrose oil

Fats That Increase Inflammation

Butter

Lamb

Beef

Roasted nuts/seeds

Dairy products

Refined oils

Margarine/trans fats

Healthy oils, such as oil from fish, hemp, or flaxseed, are rich in omega-3 fatty acids. These essential fatty acids can lower insulin levels, balance the immune system, and moderate allergic reactions.

For a more comprehensive discussion of good and bad fats, please refer to the earlier sections on eating nutritious meals and the healthy kitchen.

10. To help control inflammation, get enough sleep and manage your stress.

Stress and inflammation go hand in hand; getting enough sleep can be very helpful in controlling inflammation and balancing the immune system.

When you are sleep deprived, you are likely to experience mental fatigue, confusion, and musculoskeletal discomfort. The restorative powers of sleep and rest can bring back mental clarity and relieve various forms of stress.

How much sleep is enough? This varies by individual, particularly with regard to age, but here are some general guidelines. From the ages of sixteen to twenty-five, people need eight to nine hours of sleep to receive the full restorative benefits from it. You need less sleep as you get older. From ages twenty-five to forty-five, the need declines to seven to eight hours. Over age forty-five, people need only six to seven hours of sleep.

Rest during waking hours is also extremely helpful. In fact, sufficient daytime rest may be able to prevent stress from building up to a point where you experience problems. Meditation or guided relaxation exercises, performed for fifteen to twenty minutes twice daily, can counteract the effects of stress even if you are experiencing high levels of stress in your day-to-day work and family life.

Effective stress management can complement the healthful effects of obtaining proper rest and restoring physiological function through relaxation. Since stress causes inflammation throughout the body, you need to practice stress management techniques on a daily basis to keep the ravages of inflammation from adversely affecting your health. Refer to the earlier section on stress management for ten practical ways to reduce your stress.

Chapter Summary

Balancing your immune system is only possible with good gastrointestinal (GI) health. Injury to your GI system can imbalance your immune system and spread inflammation throughout your body, stressing your organs.

The ten recommendations described in this chapter can get you on the road to restoration of your digestive system by helping you remove harmful bacteria, yeast, and parasites; replace digestive enzymes and/or hydrochloric acid; repopulate healthy gastrointestinal bacteria; and repair the cells of your intestinal lining.

Ten Practical Ways to Balance Your Immune System

1. To improve your digestion, treat abdominal gas and bloating with digestive enzymes.
2. Restore good bacteria in your intestinal tract by taking capsules containing vibrant good bacteria.
3. Eat foods that are high in insoluble fiber to prevent constipation and eliminate toxins from intestinal tract.
4. Ingest enough soluble fiber to nourish your intestinal lining and feed good bacteria.

5. Eliminate yeast, parasites, and harmful bacteria by eating less sugar and taking specific herbs.

6. Eat whole natural foods that are very fresh—the fresher the food, the more the enzymes in the food can help you with nutrient digestion and absorption.

7. Improve gastrointestinal health with L-glutamine.

8. Follow a rotation or elimination diet to keep food allergies from causing irritation and immune imbalance.

9. Reduce inflammation by eliminating bad fats from your diet and increasing your intake of healthy fats.

10. To help control inflammation, get enough sleep and manage your stress.

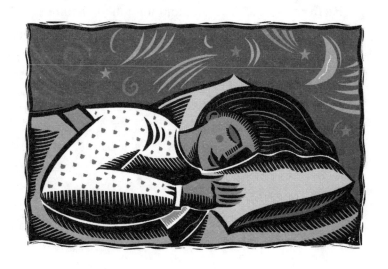

Fatigue is a result of imbalance—vitality is the reward of balance.

Key Factor Eight
Conquer Fatigue

After twenty-five years of working as a holistic, nutritionally oriented family physician, one of my most rewarding experiences is helping a new patient who has seen five or ten other physicians and still feels chronically ill.

Being a family physician doing traditional as well as alternative medicine gives me a wide range of options when dealing with individuals with chronic fatigue. Clues to the cause of your problem are hiding within your own pattern of fatigue. If you pay careful attention to these patterns, you can work with health professionals to focus on various approaches to solve the problem of your fatigue. If you take the time to follow the approaches outlined in the next three chapters, you can replicate my clinical experience of the 80 percent likelihood of restoring your full vitality.

I love changing people's lives for the better by helping them make the connections with their patterns of fatigue. I want you to live with vitality so you can create the life for which you were put on this earth.

—*Michael J. Grossman, M.D.*

Fatigue Assessment

In order to assess your level and frequency of fatigue, please answer the following questions using the scale below.

Scoring Key. Circle the number that best describes your response to each statement.

1 = never
2 = occasionally
3 = often
4 = constantly

Fatigue Assessment

My energy levels vary throughout the day.	1	2	3	4
I feel tired for hours after exercise.	1	2	3	4
I am tired every day.	1	2	3	4
I am tired on workdays but feel better on days off work.	1	2	3	4
Eating certain foods makes me tired.	1	2	3	4
I have cold hands and feet often.	1	2	3	4
I have stiffness and sore muscles not due to exercise.	1	2	3	4
My energy levels vary from day to day.	1	2	3	4

If you answered 2 to any of the above questions, you could benefit by reading this chapter.

If you answered 3 or 4 to any of the above questions, you will definitely benefit by reading this chapter.

The systems of the body can be weakened by a combination of factors including oxidative and free radical damage, poor diet, and lack of adequate nutritional supplementation. When high levels of stress or inadequate sleep are added to the mix, fatigue is a natural result. Fatigue can be described as extremely low energy resulting in a need to rest or sleep more than usual, often accompanied by headaches and body aches.

With all of the pressures we contend with in daily life, it is normal for everyone to feel some level of fatigue occasionally. When fatigue becomes a chronic problem, however, it bears watching closely to determine its causes.

Understanding Fatigue: Mitochondrial Injury

Mitochondria, which are present by the thousands in every cell of your body, are like oxygen-fueled furnaces; they convert glucose and stored fat into energy. Since the mitochondria use oxygen in energy conversion, they are very prone to the effects of oxidative stress. Your mitochondria can become injured easily through viral infection, exposure to toxins or chemicals, or an allergic reaction to medication, and the damage is difficult to repair.

Mitochondrial function can be impaired for years; this can minimize your energy level and make you more susceptible to chronic fatigue syndrome and other causes of fatigue. It can also make recovery from fatigue a more challenging and lengthy process.

Understanding Fatigue: The Adrenal Glands

The adrenal glands sit on top of the kidneys. Like the other endocrine glands, the adrenal glands are controlled by the pituitary gland. In turn, the hypothalamus, a region in the base of the brain, regulates the pituitary. This means that the brain, and in turn our emotions and thoughts, have a direct relationship to the production of stress hormones from the adrenal glands.

When you are under stress, the adrenal glands release various hormones including epinephrine, more commonly known as adrenaline, and cortisol to help you deal with stress. When the stress is chronic, the adrenal glands release a number of other hormones that cause the adrenal gland to overwork. Medical researcher Hans Selye, M.D., studied why sick people are sick and discovered a common factor: high chronic stress and adrenal gland exhaustion. After a prolonged period of hyperactivity, exhausted glands are no longer able to function at peak efficiency. At this point, you have adrenal deficiency, a cause of disabling fatigue.

Millions of adults suffer from adrenal hyperfunction, adrenal deficiency, and mitochondrial disease; but this condition, however, represents only part of the story when it comes to fatigue.

Your Fatigue Diary: Analyzing the Results

If you are experiencing chronic fatigue, whether mild or more severe, start a fatigue diary and analyze the results. Typically, you will be able to characterize your fatigue in one of four ways:

- You feel fatigue only on certain days; for example, weekdays. (#1 examines this type of fatigue.)
- You feel up and down during the day, frequently just an hour or two of feeling good or an hour or two of feeling bad. (See #2 through #4.)
- You experience fatigue only with exercise, not at rest. (See #5.)
- You feel fatigued all day, every day; your energy levels do not vary much. (See #6 through #10.)

Determine which of the four types of fatigue applies to you. After this analysis, you will be ready to put the ten recommendations described in this chapter to work to increase your energy level. Most of the therapies for treating fatigue described below allow individuals to feel much better within one to two weeks. The assumption here is that you are currently getting adequate restful sleep each night; adequate is defined by obtaining the optimum amount of sleep your body requires each night. We also assume that you experience quality sleep. If lack of sleep is your primary cause of fatigue, you might want to consider natural therapies to help you fall asleep faster and sleep more deeply, such as:

- 5-Hydroxytryptophan (5-HTP)—available through health practitioners
- Chamomile tea
- Valerian root supplements
- Melatonin supplement—0.5 to 3 mg (as you get older, your levels of melatonin decrease and you may need higher supplemental doses)
- Deep breathing techniques/meditation (see the chapter on stress reduction)

If you have difficulty breathing while lying down due to sinus problems, you should seek the advice of a physician for effective treatments to open airways.

If you do not sleep well and you wake up not feeling rested, consider getting checked for sleep apnea. If you snore you are at a high risk for sleep apnea, which is an intermittent inability to breathe in while sleeping due to the airway temporarily closing off. This can be related to being overweight as well. The diagnosis can be made by monitoring your oxygen level during the night with a finger pulse oximeter. You may need to sleep in a lab overnight for a definite diagnosis. Treatment usually means wearing a mask to increase the airway pressure in your throat. People receiving treatment for sleep apnea feel that their lives are immediately changed for the better.

Ten Practical Ways to Conquer Fatigue

1. If you experience fatigue only on workdays, find ways to manage work stress more effectively.

Your fatigue diary may reveal that you are tired only on the days you go to work, whether you work outside or inside the home. In this case, your fatigue probably has an emotional cause and is most likely related to stress on the job. On the weekends, or on days when you are not at work, you may notice that you are happier and more relaxed and do not feel as tired.

The workplace can be full of stressors, including long hours, inadequate pay, deadline pressures, and strained relationships with co-workers and management. Quitting your job is not necessarily the right answer to address stress at work. Changing your attitude, applying time management strategies, and analyzing your approach to problems can often reduce the level of stress you experience. Turn to the chapter on stress reduction for recommendations on how to more effectively manage your stress.

2. If your energy level varies during the day, test for and treat low blood sugar.

Consider low blood sugar a prime suspect if you also feel headachy, irritable, confused, nervous, or shaky along with your fatigue. The typical test for low blood sugar, a three-hour glucose tolerance test, reveals only your level of blood sugar. High insulin levels, however, may be an important player in your fatigue and present the same symptoms as low blood sugar.

To treat low blood sugar and prevent insulin surges, you need to eat high-protein foods at every meal and eat more frequent, smaller meals, five or six a day. Be sure to choose the right foods; include complex, not simple carbohydrates, as well as healthy fats. The chapter entitled Eat Balanced, Nutritious Meals contains the information you need to formulate a diet that promotes balanced levels of insulin and blood sugar.

3. If your energy level varies during the day, test for and treat adrenal gland weakness.

If you cannot get going in the morning without caffeine, adrenal gland weakness may be the culprit. Fatigue that varies through the day may be related to adrenal insufficiency. An effective treatment is to eliminate caffeine; getting beyond withdrawal symptoms takes five days. Remember that coffee is not the only dietary source of caffeine; you will also need to eliminate caffeinated tea, sodas, and chocolate. Withdrawal symptoms can include headaches; if yours are severe, you may need to reduce your intake of caffeinated beverages more gradually to moderate the withdrawal symptoms. Cut your caffeine

intake in half every three to four days until you have with-
drawn completely.

Other contributors to adrenal insufficiency include emotional and physical stress as well as low blood sugar. Helpful
supplements include vitamin B_5 or pantothenic acid, licorice
root extract, and low doses of freeze-dried adrenal gland
extract. (For recommended dosages, see Appendix C.)

4. If your energy level varies during the day, test for and treat food allergies.

Food allergies can masquerade as almost any symptom:
fatigue, body aches, joint pains, irritability, sleepiness, confusion, headaches, sore throat, itchy eyes, runny nose, coughing,
stomachaches, diarrhea, constipation, cramps, and rashes.
Ironically, if you experience strong cravings for a particular
food, it is highly likely that you are allergic to it.

Milk and wheat are the most frequently diagnosed allergens,
but peanuts, strawberries, chocolate, corn, and tomatoes also
commonly produce allergic reactions. Cooking changes the anti-
gens in vegetables, so it is possible for you to be allergic to the
cooked vegetable, but not the raw one, or vice versa.

You can determine if you have a food allergy on your own,
by experimenting with rotation diets and elimination diets and
taking careful note of physiological changes that occur with the
introduction and elimination of certain foods from your diet.
Turn to the chapter, Detoxify Your Body, for detailed information and recommendations on rotation and elimination diets.

5. If you feel fatigued only during and after exercise, treat CoQ10 deficiency.

Coenzyme Q10 (or CoQ10) is needed in the mitochondria for energy conversion and production. If your muscles do not have sufficient reserves of CoQ10, you will not be able to produce enough energy for sustained physical activity and you will fatigue easily.

You can make limited amounts of CoQ10 from the food you eat, but not necessarily all you need. In addition, as you age, you lose your ability to produce it naturally. If you are experiencing exercise-related fatigue, taking 30 to 100 mg CoQ10 twice daily can produce significant increases in your energy level.

6. If your fatigue is continual, test for and treat low thyroid.

If your fatigue is accompanied by symptoms such as cold hands and feet, constipation, weight gain, dry skin, or hoarse voice, you probably have low thyroid. Another common sign of low thyroid is low body temperature. You can test your basal body temperature by putting a thermometer under your arm first thing in the morning; a reading below 97.6 degrees can indicate low thyroid. Your physician can offer more advanced tests of thyroid levels, called free T3 and free T4, that provide much more accurate measurements than previous tests.

Thyroid glands produce two hormones, T3 and T4. T4 gets its name because it has four iodine molecules, while T3 has only three. The presence of T4 acts as a signal to the pituitary as to whether you need to produce more hormones. As we age, we become less efficient at converting T4 into the active form of T3, which involves removing a molecule of iodine. Many doctors give only T4 to patients. This is fine if the patient is young, but older patients require T3 as well.

If the results from your tests are abnormal, you may need to be treated with thyroid hormone and supplements. Selenium, a very important mineral, can support natural production of thyroid. Many people are selenium deficient and can benefit from taking selenium. The most useful thyroid supplement is desiccated animal thyroid, which contains T3 and T4.

A study published in the *New England Journal of Medicine* (April 1999) demonstrates the superior clinical results of prescribing a combination of T3 and T4 for thyroid treatment.

7. If your fatigue is continual, test for and treat vitamin B_{12} deficiency.

The majority of people over seventy years of age, as well as significant numbers of people younger than seventy, have a vitamin B_{12} deficiency. These people lose the ability to make hydrochloric acid in the stomach; the accompanying loss of a substance called intrinsic factor robs them of the ability to absorb vitamin B_{12}.

Symptoms of this deficiency include fatigue, memory loss, loss of sensation in your feet, and a loss of balance that may cause you to compensate by spreading your legs farther apart when walking. A blood test can detect this deficiency; the caveat is that the deficiency may not show up in the blood for several years. If you are suffering from these symptoms, ask your physician about a test for methylmalonic acid; this test can act as an early detection method.

Treatment involves supplementation with vitamin B_{12}. The best way to supplement is by dissolving one 1,000 mcg tablet under the tongue; by not involving your stomach, this method circumvents any problem you may have with loss of intrinsic factor. An alternative is to receive vitamin B_{12} injections; these are inexpensive and highly effective.

8. If your fatigue is continual, test for and treat anemia.

Anemia is straightforward to treat but should not be treated without first determining its cause. A simple blood test can reveal deficiencies of iron, vitamin B_{12}, and folic acid, which you can treat by taking supplements of these three nutrients. Your anemia could be caused by something as routine as menstruation; on the other hand, you could be bleeding from the gastrointestinal tract due to a colon polyp or tumor. If you are diagnosed with anemia, it is important to have an extensive medical evaluation.

9. If your fatigue is continual, test for and treat viral infections.

Any virus can cause some mitochondrial injury. Common sources of viral infection include Epstein-Barr, hepatitis B, and hepatitis C. In the case of a virus, you will need to consult a physician to undergo testing and treatment.

Unfortunately, new types of viruses are being discovered all the time, and they are all capable of damaging your immune system and your mitochondria. Medical research has revealed the insidious existence of so-called stealth viruses that masquerade as one type of virus but are in fact a completely different kind. For example, a stealth virus can incorporate into it some herpes virus DNA, and thus appear to be a herpes virus. A blood test analysis will give a false positive, showing the presence of the herpes virus. The doctor will then treat for the wrong condition (such as herpes), while the real virus goes untreated. This stealth virus also tricks your immune system, which wrongly recognizes it as herpes and ineffectively attacks it as such.

Every mother who breast feeds her infant passes on her immunity—all of the information her immune system has gained in her lifetime. This process begins with the first milk, called colostrum. The most valuable of the "immunity weapons" in colostrum are called transfer factors. The presence of transfer factor in mother's milk signals a newborn baby to turn on his or her immune system. Concentrated transfer factors can now be extracted from cow colostrum, which are available through your health practitioner. Transfer factor can boost the immune system and increase the number of killer cells available to battle bacterial and viral infections.

In addition, there are several herbal and natural immune boosters to fight viral infections, including IP6, MGM3, and mushroom extracts.

10. If your fatigue is continual, test for and treat chronic fatigue syndrome.

After close analysis, if you do not have fatigue resulting from the explanations described in #1 to #9, you probably fall into the general category of chronic fatigue syndrome. It is important to differentiate between fatigue resulting from mitochondrial injury, which is physiological, and emotional fatigue.

Chronic fatigue syndrome based on physiological injury is characterized by unexplained exhaustion and is exacerbated by any exercise or activity. If your fatigue is a result of emotional stress, not mitochondrial injury, an exercise regimen will serve as an effective course of treatment.

Frequently, there is a trigger event associated with the onset of chronic fatigue beyond stress, such as viral infection, exposure to toxins or chemicals, or an allergic reaction to medication that made you very ill and from which you never fully recovered. Long after exposure to the trigger event, chronic fatigue symptoms can persist; this is due to mitochondrial injury.

Toxicity may be a causal factor in your chronic fatigue. You can be exposed to toxic substances either externally, through heavy metals and plastics, or internally, through abnormal intestinal bacteria, leaky gut syndrome, parasites, mercury, or food allergies. It is important to explore these other avenues. See the chapters, Balance Your Immune System and Detoxify Your Body, for recommended treatment options that will help conquer fatigue resulting from toxicity.

With the right treatment for your condition, you can slowly regain your normal health. However, you will need to take good care of yourself on a permanent basis, as you will forever retain a high susceptibility to getting tired and re-injuring your mitochondria.

Chapter Summary

The high stress of daily living produces fatigue in almost everyone. The first step to eliminating fatigue is to understand when you are fatigued and why. Keeping track of every instance of fatigue in a diary will give your health professionals the information they need to treat the root causes of your exhaustion.

If you do not respond positively to any of these fatigue treatments, or if the cause remains elusive, you and your physician may want to consider other causes. One treatment course could be natural hormone therapy. Natural hormone therapy has been found to increase energy levels for a wide range of patient types and symptomology. Refer to the first chapter for information on this very effective form of treatment.

Naturally, you will need to work hand in hand with your physician to treat the root causes of your fatigue. Prescription medicines, herbs, nutrients, and glandular extracts, available from your physician, are additional treatments that may be very helpful in restoring your energy level.

Ten Practical Ways to Conquer Fatigue

If you experience fatigue only on weekdays:
1. Find ways to manage work stress.

If your fatigue level goes up and down during the day:
2. Test for and treat low blood sugar.
3. Test for and treat adrenal gland weakness.
4. Test for and treat food allergies.

If you feel fatigued only during and after exercise:
5. Treat CoQ10 deficiency.

If your fatigue is continual:
6. Test for and treat low thyroid.
7. Test for and treat vitamin B_{12} deficiency.
8. Test for and treat anemia.
9. Test for and treat viral infections.
10. Test for and treat chronic fatigue syndrome.

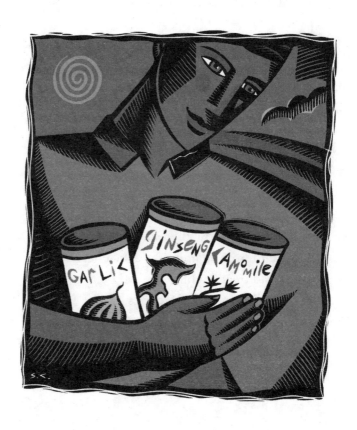

It's not easy abstaining from cravings—discipline is the foundation for optimized detoxification.

Key Factor Nine
Detoxify Your Body

My interest in food allergies and detoxification began in medical school when I heard on a radio show about "the food allergy–addiction syndrome." I was addicted to bread and cream cheese. When I tried abstaining, I got headaches and became irritable and fatigued. Then, for the first time in my life, I made a connection between eating specific foods and my experiences with low energy, headaches, body aches, and rashes.

I have treated thousands of patients with food allergy programs. I believe that food allergies are a major factor in chronic illness, fatigue, headaches, rashes, and intestinal upsets, as well as learning disabilities, autism, and a myriad of other symptoms.

What makes dealing with food allergies so rewarding is how quickly people respond. Within two weeks people consistently notice great improvements.

Please use this section as an opportunity to learn how to detoxify your body from the buildup of residues, immune complexes, and toxins that relate to chronic illness.

—Michael J. Grossman, M.D.

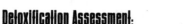

Detoxification Assessment:

In order to assess your potential toxicity, please answer the following questions with a "yes" or "no."

Detoxification Assessment

I become ill around perfume, paint smells, or cigarette smoke.
I have silver dental fillings.
I have less than one bowel movement daily.
I crave certain foods daily such as dairy, wheat, sugar, and so on.
I do not feel full until I eat certain foods.
I feel best if I do not eat at all.
I do not feel well after eating certain foods.
I get sleepy after eating.
I eat tuna, swordfish, and shark more than once per month.
I use a shower without a water filter.
I eat fried fast foods or foods that contain partially hydrogenated oils.
I experience joint pains or osteoarthritis.
I eat dark green leafy vegetables less than three times weekly.

If you answered yes to any the above questions, you will benefit by reading this chapter.

Since World War II, over seventy thousand different synthetic chemicals have been developed for use in foods, cosmetics, fertilizers, pesticides, and other products. While federal agencies such as the U.S. Department of Agriculture (USDA), Occupational Safety and Health Administration (OSHA), and Environmental Protection Agency (EPA) have attempted to monitor and evaluate these chemicals, only a small fraction (less than 15 percent) have been extensively studied. Complicating matters, over one thousand new chemical substances are developed each year.[1]

The consequences of toxic exposure can include skin irritation, birth defects, cancer, cardiovascular disease, respiratory problems, neurological disorders, predisposition to genetic (DNA) injury, allergies, depletion of stored antioxidants, autoimmune disorders, and even death. It is estimated that men and women born in the 1940s have a 35 percent greater chance of contracting cancer than their grandparents did.

Over six billion pounds of toxic substances are released into the environment each year.[2] These substances find their way into the food supply, the water supply, and the soil, harming you and your family. Unfortunately, such contamination is often very difficult to detect and the first indication may come with a decline in your health.

These toxins represent a burden on your body from external sources, but this alone is not the complete picture. To survive and thrive, you must not only neutralize the effects of external toxins, but also render harmless an equal challenge of internal toxins produced, stored, and periodically released within the body.

Understanding Detoxification

Detoxification can be defined as eliminating toxic buildup from your body; internal toxins are created from by-products of the foods that you eat and your own metabolic processes. A toxin is basically any substance that creates irritating and/or harmful effects in the body, undermining health and stressing biochemical or organ function.

General detoxification systems include:

- Gastrointestinal—liver, gallbladder, colon, and the entire GI tract
- Urinary—kidneys, bladder, and urethra
- Respiratory—lungs, bronchial tubes, throat, sinuses, and nose
- Lymphatic—lymph channels and lymph nodes
- Skin—sweat, sebaceous glands, and tears

Detoxification begins when toxic substances in the blood enter the liver. These substances must be made water soluble before they can pass out through the kidneys. This is a two-phase process. Phase I makes these fat-soluble substances partially water soluble; Phase II makes them water soluble to the point where the toxin can be completely excreted from the body in the urine. [3]

Any toxic substances that are not processed through detoxification in the liver get pushed back into the bloodstream, from which they may enter the liver later for a subsequent attempt at detoxification, or are stored in fat, brain, or nervous system cells. Your fat cells, for example, may contain stored DDT, prescription medicines, antibiotics, pollutants, plastics, contaminants, estrogenic substances, mercury and other heavy metals, trans fats, and by-products of yeast metabolism.

Some people are not efficient at detoxification due to their genetic makeup, and the result is increasing amounts of toxic buildup. Such people with unbalanced or slow detoxifying systems may be more likely to suffer from a variety of conditions, including headaches, fibromyalgia, chronic fatigue, rashes, body aches and pains, and digestive problems. [4-7] Despite the role genetics plays in this ability to detoxify, healthy choices can make all the difference.

Detoxification is a process that can benefit any person when it is done safely, thoughtfully, and with the proper supervision.[8] It is important to detoxify/cleanse for health, vitality, and rejuvenation. It can help clear symptoms, treat disease, and prevent future problems. A cleansing program is an effective way to help reevaluate our lives, make more healthful choices, clear abuses, and reduce addictions. The ten recommendations that follow will provide safe and effective suggestions for detoxification.

Ten Practical Ways to Detoxify Your Body

1. **Obtain medical testing to benchmark your levels of toxicity. Testing can also reveal the relative effectiveness or ineffectiveness of your body, in particular the liver, in processing and neutralizing toxins.**

   For genetic reasons, some people are more successful than others at cleaning out injurious substances and toxins. Testing can determine whether you are a fast, slow, or unbalanced detoxifier. If you are an unbalanced detoxifier who is efficient and effective during Phase I detoxification and much slower during Phase II, you face the highest risk for toxic buildup in the liver. Testing will point out your toxic risk and reveal how important it may be for you to institute lifestyle changes to combat toxic buildup.

   There are various tests that are useful in analyzing your toxicity levels and detoxification capabilities. The following three are very effective tests: bioimpedence analysis (BIA), biological terrain analysis (BTA), and measuring homocysteine levels through blood tests.

BIA testing measures inflammation and resultant puffiness by calculating the ratio of intracellular versus extracellular water. The body has a certain balance it likes to maintain; when it cannot maintain this state any longer, the body develops puffiness, particularly in the hands and feet. When people are allergic or sensitive to certain foods they find they experience this puffiness and bloating. The healthiest condition is to have at least 60 percent of your total body water inside the cells.

As you become less healthy and encounter increasing levels of inflammation, the ratio of extracellular to intracellular water will rise. When your liver does not succeed in removing all the toxins sent its way, the remaining toxins go back into the extracellular water. Toxins accumulate in the extracellular water and then journey to the liver for detoxification.

The cells continually monitor the level of toxicity in the extracellular water; when toxicity levels get too high, the cells respond by excreting water from within to dilute the toxin-rich extracellular water. This is a vicious cycle that results in further imbalance.

Biological terrain analysis (BTA) is a computerized analysis of blood, saliva, and urine that provides a wealth of information about your internal terrain or biochemistry. If you are too acidic or too alkaline, your body's enzymes cannot function effectively. BTA reveals whether digestion and absorption of vitamins, minerals, and nutrients are occurring properly. Levels of toxicity are assessed. Also, oxidative stress levels are measured directly.

Mineral concentration can be too low, indicating deficiency in nutritional absorption. Overly concentrated minerals suggest congestion and stagnation of vital dynamic body fluids. After treatment with nutrition, vitamins, minerals, herbs, homeopathy, and exercises, repeat testing will indicate whether the treatments are effectively improving your biochemistry. When your body does not have enough vitamin B_{12}, B_6, folic acid and required cofactors for reduction of homocysteine levels, homocysteine can become a toxic substance. High levels may cause acute injury to your arteries and your brain, and even trigger the onset of Alzheimer's disease, nerve injury, and DNA injury.

Homocysteine is elevated in about 20 percent of Americans. A quick look at the disease progeria can provide a vivid demonstration of how elevated homocysteine can accelerate the aging process. Progeria is a rare medical condition in which small children, genetically unable to reduce their homocysteine levels, look and feel as old as a very elderly person. In many cases of progeria, patients do not survive into their teenage years.

2. Avoid using water or juice fasts to detoxify.

Subsisting on water or fruit juice for a full day or longer can be dangerous. You need to take in healthy calories every day; if your daily intake falls below 800 calories, your body starts consuming not only fat but also muscle and protein.

Burning your own body fat can be hazardous in itself. Chemicals and pesticides are stored in fat permanently, until released. When you minimize caloric intake during a fast, your body turns to your fat stores for fuel. The toxic chemicals,

DDT and other pesticides, and heavy metals that are stored in your fat cells will be released directly into your bloodstream and can cause powerful negative reactions.

Recommendation #3 provides information about how to keep your daily intake above the 800-calorie threshold. This includes consuming conventional meals and medically based foods that can aid in the detoxification process.[9–11]

3. When following a detoxification diet, consume food and powdered medically based foods that optimize the detoxification process.

There are medically based detoxification beverage mixes available through nutrition-focused doctors that contain supplements and nutrients that help your body to detoxify. (See Appendix F for recommendations.) These detoxification drinks offer the necessary vitamins and minerals, including B vitamins, folic acid, minerals, selenium, zinc, and antioxidants, to defend against stress to your liver.[12] Sulfur compounds and amino acids, such as glycine and taurine, are added to support effective Phase II detoxification. As part of a detoxification diet, many physicians have their patients consume three to five servings daily of a detoxification drink to give the liver the extra nutritional support it needs.

Alkaline Broth Recipe

Below is a recipe for an alkaline broth that will help you detoxify during the first few days of a detoxification diet.

Place equal amounts of the following vegetables in a steamer basket: spinach, zucchini, parsley, celery, and green beans. Make sure that the steamer basket remains above the level of the water at all times. Steam the vegetables, testing them with a fork to ensure that they do not become soft. Remove the vegetables from the steamer while still crunchy. Place the vegetables and the water in which you steamed them into a blender. Puree the mixture in the blender, adding your favorite herbs (such as basil, garlic, or dill) for flavor. Drink eight ounces of this alkaline broth for the first few days during detoxification.

To promote liver health, there are effective herbal supplements such as milk thistle, also known as silymarin. Silymarin selectively acts as an antioxidant and protects from free radical damage specifically in the intestines, liver, and stomach. It increases the liver's content of glutathione, a substance that detoxifies many potentially damaging hormones, chemicals, and certain drugs, including acetaminophen.

4. Use a rotation diet or elimination diet as a method for detecting food sensitivities and to clear your body of accumulated toxins.

If you have previously read the chapter, Balancing Your Immune System, you are already familiar with some of the concepts behind rotation and elimination diets. Using this diet for detoxification purposes requires restrictive procedures regarding how and when foods are rotated back into the diet.

Foods to which you have sensitivities are toxic to your body and your body has only limited success at processing these foods. Since it takes about four days for you to resolve a reaction to a given food, you need to plan and shop for your meals carefully so that you do not eat the same food any more frequently than once every four days.

To follow a program specifically for detoxification, start by eliminating these common food allergens for an initial period of two weeks:

- Wheat and other glutens
- Dairy
- Beef
- Peanuts
- Chocolate
- Caffeine, including caffeinated coffee, tea, and soft drinks
- Sugar

Withdrawal from allergenic foods can produce symptoms similar to those a drug addict or alcoholic may experience. Initially, you may feel headaches, nausea, and other discomfort due to withdrawal from allergenic foods and caffeine; these ill effects should disappear completely within five days.

Throughout the first week, eat fresh fruits every day but rotate them on a daily basis. Choose from pears, apricots, plums, papaya, mango, grapes, and berries other than strawberries; since many people are allergic to strawberries, we suggest you avoid these. Eat lightly steamed vegetables and drink the alkaline broth (see recipe in #3). The best choices are low-starch, high–water content vegetables such as celery, green beans, broccoli, cabbage, brussel sprouts, and zucchini. After four days, you should begin to add healthy fats; use small amounts, one teaspoon of extra virgin olive oil, flaxseed oil, or sesame oil.

Throughout the entire period you are on the diet, be sure to eat five small meals daily. In fact, this is a sound lifestyle choice to implement and maintain as a lifelong dietary habit.

Small, frequent meals will help you avoid feeling hungry and will give your digestive system a lighter workload than when you eat a small number of large, more heavy meals. Your body will require adequate supplies of water to aid in detoxification; be sure to drink eight or more glasses of pure filtered water daily.

For a specific list of which foods to eat and those to avoid, please see Appendix F.

5. Record everything you eat in a diary and note your reactions to each food. Use your diary to guide you as you begin to rotate foods back into your diet.

As you complete the first week of the diet, it is time to begin step-by-step rotation of foods back into your diet. You may notice that you are feeling dramatically better at this point; this is the result of eliminating food allergens from your diet and allowing your body to gradually detoxify substances that have accumulated in your system. As you add back in foods you have eliminated, be sure to note any food reactions in your diary.

Gradually adding back foods requires considerable patience and self-control; this process is critical to identifying your individual food allergies and sensitivities. Certain foods, particularly those that produce acute reactions every single time you eat them, will have to be permanently eliminated from your diet. On the other hand, your diary may help you single out some foods, even ones that are quite allergenic to your system, that produce negative reactions only when eaten frequently, two times a week or more. By keeping careful track of these foods in your diary, you may discover that you are able to eat these foods once every four days without experiencing a significant reaction.

Check the diary for your food reactions during the first week. If you have not noticed any reactions to the fruits, you may begin eating more than one fruit per day. If you are feeling well at the seven-day mark, start introducing the following foods, and observe your reactions to these foods:

- Rice, millet, and buckwheat
- Cold-water fish such as salmon, cod, and sardines
- Eggs, preferably free range or eggs that are high in omega-3 fats. (The healthiest method of preparation is poaching.)
- Chicken and turkey, baked or broiled, not fried.
- Legumes (beans), raw nuts, and seeds.

If you have not yet become an avid label reader, now is a great time to acquire the habit. Food additives and preservatives can also produce powerful reactions in the body. Scrutinize package labels carefully for substances such as phosphates, aluminum, monosodium glutamate, nitrates, and preservatives.

6. Learn the facts about foods that help or hinder the liver in detoxification. Do not add back into your diet any foods that may impede detoxification.

Long-term detoxification requires total elimination of bad fats, since they cause inflammation throughout the body. Examples of bad fats include shortening, margarine, and partially hydrogenated oil; products that typically include trans-fatty acids (trans fats) are baked goods, fried foods, candies, and potato chips—nearly all snack "junk" foods.

Trans fats act as toxins in the body; they injure the cell walls, confuse cell transport mechanisms, and accumulate within the cells. They have a similar effect in the brain, where they can hasten the onset of Alzheimer's disease and other disorders.

Good fats, called omega-3 fats, are found in fish, flaxseeds, and hemp seeds. Olive and canola oil also fall into the category of good fats. For a further discussion of good fats, please refer to the chapter, Eat Balanced Nutritious Meals.

Two other common substances conflict with the detoxification process and merit special mention because they suppress liver enzymes. One is the over-the-counter remedy Tagamet (cimetidine), used to relieve heartburn and acid indigestion. The other is grapefruit juice. It is not necessary to eliminate grapefruit juice entirely, just do not drink it daily. On the other hand, it is better not to use Tagamet at all, especially considering the wide availability of other effective over-the-counter medications that perform the same function, such as Zantac (ranitidine) and Pepcid (famotidine).

7. Avoid storing beverages or foods in plastic containers, and keep plastic containers away from sources of heat.

Try to reduce your use of plastics. Plastic containers, cookware, and kitchen accessories, especially when heated, can leach out substances that are toxic and extremely estrogenic. For this reason, use glass instead of plastic in the microwave and do not leave water bottles exposed in your car on a warm day; the extreme heat will initiate this toxic leaching process.

Plastic manufacturers, guided by consumer preferences and the bottom line, have actually increased the toxicity of containers in recent decades. The goal of the manufacturers has been to make plastics more and more flexible, and they have succeeded at making products that are extremely inexpensive and unbreakable. However, when you heat up these plastic products, they release compounds that the body recognizes as a super estrogen. These estrogenic properties may contribute to hormonal imbalance over time. To help neutralize the side effects of heated plastic, you can take a supplement called Indole-3-Carbinol (I3C). This is a nutrient derived from cauliflower and broccoli that will allow your body to metabolize estrogens safely.

8. Reduce your exposure to heavy metals, such as aluminum and mercury. Small doses of selenium can aid your body in excreting, rather than absorbing, mercury.

The chapter on a healthy kitchen includes discussion of the safest tools for cooking. Stock your kitchen with cookware made of stainless steel, glass, or stoneware; avoid cast iron and aluminum. Aluminum is so soft that when it is heated, toxic metal compounds can leach into the food as you cook.

Mercury also creates significant toxicity problems. Unfortunately, the oceans and the fish supply contain large amounts of mercury. The problem is amplified in the case of large fish, such as swordfish, shark, and tuna, which eat other smaller fish, therefore resulting in compounded mercury consumption. Your safest choices are small fish such as sardines and farm-raised fish. Fish that are farm raised do not contain mercury, since what these fish eat can be strictly controlled.

You can protect yourself against toxic buildup caused by eating fish. Within thirty minutes after consuming fish, take at least 50 mcg of selenium. The selenium will bind with the mercury, and the toxins will be excreted through the stool rather than absorbed into your body.

9. Purchase organic foods to reduce toxic buildup.

Foods that are labeled organic are grown with virtually no pesticides and chemical fertilizers. Thankfully, there is now enough demand for organic produce that you may not have to make a special trip to the health food store for it; many large grocery store chains stock organic fruits and vegetables in their produce departments. Animal products may also be labeled organic; for example, you can buy organic milk produced by cows that have not been given doses of bovine growth hormone and organic and free-range eggs from chickens that have not been exposed to high levels of hormones or pesticides in their feed.

Pesticides can be hazardous to your health because they build up in your body and can be stored in your fat until released. When you lose weight, burning of fat can suddenly release dangerous substances into your bloodstream and cause toxicity problems. Over the years, pesticides build up in your body and may even eventually cause cancer.

10. Take steps to minimize your daily exposure to environmental toxins from drinking water and bath/shower water.

The introduction to this chapter discusses some of the sources of environmental contaminants that contribute to the high levels of toxicity experienced by people living in industrialized nations. With all these external environmental toxins to contend with, it is wise to minimize your risks by eliminating sources of contaminants when possible.

In a single year, six billion pounds of chemicals, released by natural means as well as illegal dumping, filter down into the water table and make ordinary tap water into a potentially hazardous material. Many people, having become aware of this fact, have responded by making the switch to bottled drinking water or by installing water purification systems. However, what you drink is only part of the problem; you can also absorb chemical contaminants in the water supply through your skin.

One way to avoid taking in toxins through your skin is to install a charcoal filter in your shower. An attachment that uses another filtering process, reverse osmosis, is fine for the sink, but you will not be able to get adequate water pressure if you use a reverse osmosis filter in the shower. Charcoal does not choke off your water pressure and is much better suited for shower use.

Chapter Summary

Every day you must neutralize external toxins and pollutants as well as toxic substances produced within the body. By making the healthy choices advised in these ten recommendations, you can dramatically improve your body's ability to detoxify itself. This chapter describes measures of toxicity, specific detoxification diets, and fasting with detoxification powdered nutritional food supports. The rotation and elimination diets are critical parts of a detoxification program.

Ten Practical Ways to Detoxify Your Body

1. Obtain medical testing to benchmark your levels of toxicity. Testing can also reveal the relative effectiveness or ineffectiveness of your body, in particular the liver, in processing and neutralizing toxins.

2. Avoid using water or juice fasts to detoxify.

3. When following a detoxification diet, consume food and powdered foods that optimize the detoxification process.

4. Use a rotation diet or elimination diet as a method for detecting food sensitivities and to clear your body of accumulated toxins.

5. Record everything you eat in a diary, and note your reactions to each food. Use your diary to guide you as you begin to rotate foods back into your diet.

6. Learn the facts about foods that help or hinder the liver in detoxification. Do not add back into your diet any foods that may impede detoxification.

7. Avoid storing beverages or foods in plastic containers, and keep plastic containers away from sources of heat.

8. Reduce your exposure to heavy metals, such as aluminum and mercury. Small doses of selenium can aid your body in excreting, rather than absorbing, toxic heavy metals.

9. Purchase organic foods to reduce toxic buildup.

10. Take steps to minimize your daily exposure to environmental toxins from drinking water and bath/shower water.

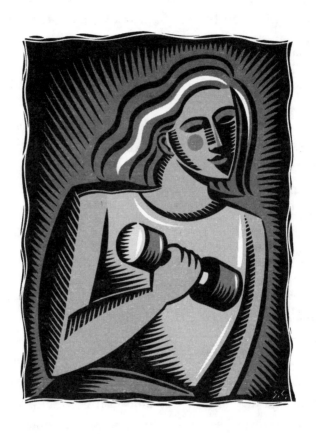

Without moderate exercise, it is not possible to have a successful anti-aging program.

Key Factor Ten
Commit to an Exercise Program

I have always had a love/hate relationship with exercise. I loved how it reshaped my body, but I hated taking the time and energy to work out. In my teens and twenties, my vanity and social interests motivated most of my exercising. In my thirties, as my autoimmune diseases progressed, I found the perfect excuse to not work out anymore; it was far too painful and I certainly didn't have the energy to do all that work.

Now, in my forties, I am much better informed and mature enough to realize the true benefits of and value from a consistent and moderate exercise regimen. Without a balanced cardiovascular and strength-training program, my progress toward recovery would not have been possible. I don't have the discipline to maximize my workouts on my own, so I have a personal trainer who keeps me focused and on track to achieve my health and fitness goals.

One of the best things you can do for disease prevention, stress release, increased energy, and overall emotional and physical well-being is exercise. Whether you use a personal trainer to get you jump-started or are self-motivated and disciplined, as the commercial says, "Just Do It!"

—Jodi L. Jones

In terms of wellness and longevity, diet, exercise, and stress management are very closely related. Vigorous or moderate exercise accompanied by poor dietary habits and high levels of stress is no more effective in reversing the aging process than is a complete lack of exercise accompanied by healthy dietary habits and low levels of stress. To maximize vitality, it is critical to embrace all three disciplines: proper diet, consistent exercise, and stress management. For optimum gain, it is important to split your exercise training time among the various types of exercise described in this chapter.

The benefits of exercise go beyond slowing down the aging process. Consistent exercise can lower insulin resistance, balance hormone levels, build muscle mass, reduce fat, increase energy and endurance, build strength, improve flexibility, prevent disease, reduce the risk for osteoporosis, reduce stress, promote psychological well-being, and improve overall self-image. It is clear that basically everyone can reap significant benefits from a regular fitness regime, those who already appear physically fit and those who do not.

The heart is a muscle, and exercise strengthens it. With exercise, the heart can produce more powerful contractions and pump the blood around the body more effectively. Exercise, combined with proper diet and stress management, is critical for changing or maintaining hormonal balance and helps prevent and reverse the hormonal changes that cause Type 2 diabetes, high blood pressure, high cholesterol, obesity, and arthritis. Exercise also increases your metabolic rate, so that you burn more calories at rest and do not store as many of the excess calories you consume as fat.

The approach you take toward fitness contributes a great deal to the success you will experience. Improving your fitness level is not a sprint; it is a contest of endurance. Slow and steady progress day by day is the most important factor for success. Getting off to a fast start, only to burn out and quit later, creates no lasting health benefits.

Types of Exercises

Aerobic Exercise

Aerobic means "with oxygen." Because aerobic exercise requires oxygen from the air to get to your muscles, the exercise can continue only when a source of oxygen is available. Your heart and lungs work together to supply oxygen to tissues in your body. Aerobic exercise forces the lungs and heart to work harder and, in so doing, strengthens and conditions them.

Aerobic activities include walking, bicycling, lap swimming, aqua aerobics (low-impact and low-intensity water therapy, ideal for arthritis sufferers and the elderly), jogging, singles tennis, basketball, and cross-country skiing. The minute you start to exercise, your metabolic rate (the amount of energy you expend) immediately increases to somewhere between five and twenty times what you expend sitting down. This change is very health promoting when it takes place on a regular basis.

Anaerobic Exercise

Anaerobic means "without oxygen." An anaerobic exercise is any exercise that requires short bursts of power, such as all-out sprinting or very heavy weight lifting, which does not require a significant increase in oxygen delivery to the muscle. The ability to perform this type of work is dependent instead on energy sources stored in the muscle. Anaerobic exercise can be sustained for only short periods of time because this energy supply is limited. In reality, most exercise is a combination of aerobic and anaerobic exercise. The amount of each is dependent on how hard and fast the exercise proceeds.

Resistance Exercise

Resistance exercise, also called strength training, increases muscle strength and mass, bone strength, and metabolic rate. It can also help you maintain or lose weight and improve your body image.

Methods for resistance training include free weights, weight machines, and calisthenics. A newer form of resistance training involves the use of an elastic band, called resistance tubing, that provides resistance to the active muscles.

Isometric Exercise

In this type of strength-training exercise, your muscles contract, but your joints do not move and your muscle fibers maintain a constant length. The exercises are typically performed against an immovable surface; for example, pressing your palm against a wall. Isometric training is effective for developing total strength of a particular muscle or group of muscles. It is often used for rehabilitation because the exact area of muscle weakness can be isolated and strengthening exercises can be administered at the proper joint angle.

Isotonic and Isokinetic Exercise

In isotonic exercise, a body part is moved and the muscle shortens or lengthens. Although sit-ups, push-ups and pull-ups are isotonic, lifting free weights, such as dumbbells and barbells, is considered the classic form of isotonic exercise.

Flexibility Exercise

Flexibility exercises use gentle stretching movements to increase the length of your muscle fibers and the effective range of motion in your joints. They may consist of a series of specific stretching exercises, or be part of a larger exercise program such as yoga or dance classes. Since one of the main goals of stretching is to lengthen the connective tissue surrounding your muscle fibers, flexibility exercises should be done after you have already warmed up your muscles with a few minutes of aerobic activity.

Gain without Pain

The common exercise expression states, "No pain, no gain." This is somewhat of a myth. There are no benefits conferred by extreme pain from flexibility and aerobic exercise. Certain specific types of pain, such as muscle aches and soreness twenty-four to forty-eight hours after a weight-lifting session, are to be expected. In fact, if soreness is not experienced, you can conclude that you did not build new muscle. However, stabbing pain in your shoulder, elbow, or knee is more likely to be a sign of injury. If you experience severe pain, stop immediately and take off enough time from training to recover and heal. Avoiding overtraining is one of the keys to long-term fitness success.

When exercising, listen to your body. It is very easy to get excited about the benefits exercise will bring you, and during the early stages, many people push themselves too hard too fast for their fitness level. If you find yourself getting sick or injured more frequently at the start of your exercise program or during periods of heavy training, your body is trying to tell you to slow down a little. Excessively sore or stiff muscles are one sign of overtraining. Here are several others:

- Increases in resting blood pressure or heart rate
- Loss of coordination
- Irritability
- Decreases in appetite
- Decreases in muscle strength
- Decline in physical performance

Safeguard your health by consulting with a medical practitioner before beginning any exercise program. If your personal or family medical history includes such conditions as cardiovascular disease, diabetes, high blood pressure, or discomfort or shortness of breath during or following exercise, this is not just a precaution; it is a medical necessity. You will find more discussion of the role of health professionals in your fitness regimen in the ten recommendations that follow.

Ten Practical Ways to Commit to an Exercise Program

1. **Before beginning your regimen, identify your exercise goals and objectives. To guide you in designing your exercise program and tracking your progress, see a medical practitioner to obtain a physical exam and baseline medical information.**

People begin exercise programs for a variety of reasons: weight loss, toning, increasing strength and flexibility, and improving cardiovascular function. All these are important, and exercise accelerates progress in each of these areas.

Discuss your goals and objectives with your licensed health practitioner and obtain medical advice regarding your proposed program. Undergo a stress EKG every two years over the age of forty to be sure that exercise is safe for you and that you are not developing heart disease.

A health practitioner can also conduct physiological age scoring. Refer to #2 in the first chapter on anti-aging for more information. Scoring your physiological versus chronological age gives you information on your health, including percentage of body fat, percentage of muscle mass, and muscle strength. This assessment provides a baseline you and your health practitioner can utilize in tracking your progress throughout the year.

Your health practitioner, as well as an exercise physiologist or experienced personal trainer, can also identify your target heart rate zone to monitor throughout any cardiovascular training workout. For information on how to calculate your target heart rate zone by yourself, see #6 below, which discusses cardiovascular training.

2. Assess how self-motivated you are. This will determine how you can best maximize the success of your fitness program through the services of a personal trainer, fitness club, or home gym.

The first two months of training, when you establish good exercise habits, are the hardest, and your success during this period is critical to your decision about whether to continue with your program. If you do not have the necessary knowledge on how to exercise to produce maximum benefits and prevent injury, you are probably not a good candidate for a do-it-yourself approach.

Your choice of how to train—in a home gym, at a fitness club, or with a personal trainer—should be based on how self-motivated you are and how much external motivation you may need to keep yourself on track.

- **Home gym.** A home gym may be the ideal choice for you if you are very self-motivated and have the money to spend on the right equipment. Busy professionals generally respond well to the unmatched convenience of a home gym; for these people, time is money, and they are able to work out without having to commute to a club, which can save thirty to sixty minutes or more per workout. Even if there are adverse weather conditions such as a blizzard or tornado, your workout equipment is always close at hand if there is a gym set up in your home.

  Expense is definitely a factor for those who choose this method. You may need several pieces of costly equipment to get a well-rounded workout: one for cardiovascular training such as a stationary bike, stair stepper, or elliptical trainer, and equipment for weight training, including barbells and free weights, or a weight machine with multiple stations. You may even wish to purchase a workout video or two to help keep you motivated and make your workouts feel less solitary and more social.

■ **Fitness club.** A fitness club may not be as convenient as a home gym, but it does not require an investment in home equipment. A fitness club also offers a wide range of equipment to use and aerobic- and cardio-training classes led by professional instructors.

Joining a fitness club also involves some expense, but the competitiveness of this industry enables prospective members to purchase memberships at low cost. Check the ads in the sports page and/or health section of your newspaper to see if there are any special deals available.

Tour the club beforehand to make sure it offers varied workouts and the right equipment for your program and is not so crowded that working out there involves too much hassle, extra time, and aggravation. Do a little detective work to determine if there are long lines in front of the machines you want to use at your favorite workout times and if parking is hard to come by during peak hours. Are benefits such as classes, a swimming pool, basketball and racquetball courts, towel service, lockers, and child care included in your monthly fees, or do they require an additional payment or upgraded membership?

Some clubs offer a limited-time "try before you buy" membership. Most commercial fitness clubs offer some kind of orientation or consultation with a staff trainer as a complimentary extra included with your membership, or will include a free consultation as an incentive to get you to sign up. During this free consultation, the staff trainer can set up a complete fitness program for you, as well as show you how to use all the necessary equipment.

Give some thought to location before making a membership commitment. A club that is near your office may enable you to sneak in a workout during lunch or downtime, while a club near home is more convenient on the weekends. A club located somewhere in the middle may be the best of both worlds.

For those who are motivated by being around other people working out and enjoy the social aspect, joining a fitness club might be the best choice. The goal is to make a decision based on what will keep you motivated and on track.

- **Personal trainer.** If setting up regular appointments with a personal trainer will make exercise a firm commitment in your schedule and help maintain your motivation, it is well worth the expense and effort to locate a certified trainer in your area. Establishing an effective program from the start, and learning how to perform the exercises correctly, will save you a lot of time and money and help prevent injuries. Personal trainers offer a combination of personalized attention, professional expertise, and motivation that is difficult to attain on your own.

  When searching for a personal trainer, bear in mind that their viewpoints can vary greatly; look for one that is in sync with your own training philosophy and also has the right educational background, certifications, communication skills, experience level, fee structure, and billing and cancellation policies. Make sure that the trainer has ample appointment slots open at workout times that are the most convenient for you. Ask for client references and check them out; then, ask yourself if the trainer's approach and personality will allow the two of you to get along well. You need to find someone whose personal style will motivate you to keep your workout appointments instead of finding excuses to cancel or postpone them.

An ideal solution is a personal trainer who works at a small private gym. This way you get the advantages of having an expert guide you through your exercise program and the benefit of using various types of fitness equipment without experiencing the long waits typically associated with larger fitness clubs.

3. Work with a certified professional trainer to establish a fitness routine appropriate for your health conditions and fitness objectives.

Even if you do not intend to use the services of a trainer over the long term, it is very wise to begin your program by obtaining an initial consultation. If you join a club, this service may be included in your membership.

A certified professional trainer can advise you regarding types of exercises, quantity, repetitions, amount of weight, rotation, and a host of other important factors with which you may be unfamiliar. For example, a good program will include exercises that work all of the major muscle groups; if you try to design your own program without a solid knowledge of human physiology, your program may be not as comprehensive as it should be, and it may yield incomplete benefits.

Obtaining the services of a certified trainer does not require a long-term commitment. The objective of this initial consultation is to make sure you are performing the exercises correctly before you actually do your body more harm than good.

4. Be consistent with your exercise routine. Work out a minimum of three days per week for at least forty-five minutes.

There are several different types of workouts for you to complete each week: cardiovascular, upper-body strengthening, lower-body strengthening, and flexibility stretching. That is a lot of training for you to accomplish in three sessions per week.

Packing everything into three sessions each week requires you to do each type of exercise in every workout. That is why working out five days a week is ideal. This higher frequency permits workout rotation, promotes variety, maintains your interest and motivation, lessens the degree of muscle soreness you may experience, and shortens the duration of each workout. You can alternate muscle groups if you work out more than three times a week: work on lower-body strengthening one day, then switch to upper-body strengthening in your next workout.

5. Warm up for at least ten minutes before every workout.

A proper warm-up is essential for many reasons. Warming up your muscles may prevent injuries and increase muscle efficiency for the workout to come; it may also enhance neuromuscular coordination and increase oxygen reserves in the muscles. For best results from your workout, your muscles and joints need at least a ten-minute warm-up before exerting any pressure or force.

A medium-paced walk, either outside or on a treadmill, in which you keep your arms in constant motion, is a reliable warm-up technique. For best results, never skip your warm up.

6. Devote a significant portion of your workout time to cardiovascular training.

Cardiovascular, or aerobic training produces tremendous health benefits. Aerobic exercise reduces stress and relaxes the cardiovascular system. Cardio training includes indoor activities such as using a treadmill, stair climber, or rowing machine; kickboxing; and aerobic dancing. It also includes outdoor activities, such as swimming, biking, and walking. Many outdoor activities that contribute to cardiovascular fitness require no special equipment or trips to a fitness club. These activities offer opportunities to increase endurance; you can choose to run in sand along the beach, for example, or walk up hills instead of sticking to flat terrain.

After just six weeks of training three or more times per week, you will feel invigorated rather than exhausted following your workout; you will have enhanced energy and vitality and be better able to manage stress. If, however, you feel fatigued after working out on a regular basis, refer to the recommendations in the chapter, Conquer Fatigue.

The Importance of Your Target Zone

Any discussion of cardiovascular training must include the concept of the target heart rate zone. Your maximum heart rate is the theoretical maximum number of times your heart can beat in a minute. You can estimate your maximum heart rate by subtracting your age from 220. For example, 220 minus 40 years of age equals a maximum heart rate of 180. This is a commonly used formula for the average person but is only accurate for about 75 percent of the population, as it does not take into consideration resting heart rate or oxygen consumption and utilization, which varies greatly for each person.

There are more specific, clinical formulas used by trained doctors and exercise physiologists to obtain more accurate rates, such as the Karvonen formula that factors in resting heart rate, or using VO_2 (oxygen consumption, transport, and utilization). The latter method is used primarily for highly trained athletes.

During aerobic training, the goal is to keep your heart rate in the target heart rate zone for a minimum of twenty minutes, and ideally up to sixty minutes. The target heart rate zone ranges from 55 percent for a minimally fit person to 90 percent for conditioned athletes. For example, for a minimally fit forty-year-old, the approximate target heart rate zone would be 99 beats per minute (55 percent of 180 equals 99). If you are starting your exercise program as a beginner who is in poor shape, stay close to this range, or even a bit below, to avoid overexertion. People in better shape can exercise safely at higher points in their target zones. You can monitor your heart rate during exercise by manually checking your pulse, or by using a sensor that measures your heart rate. Some cardiovascular fitness machines even have heart rate monitors built right into the unit.

Generally speaking, if you are not sweating, you are not pushing yourself enough. Even when you are not doing cardio training on a given day, engaging in a twenty-minute brisk walk is ideal when combined with a three-day weekly routine of more intense cardio in your target heart rate zone.

Variety is just as important in cardiovascular training as it is in other forms of exercise. Alternate between a handful of activities you enjoy: swim one day, bike the next, then go for a brisk walk or jog, or even take up karate or another form of physical training. Each exercise works different muscle groups and helps keep your motivation high.

7. Devote a significant portion of your workout time to strength training.

As late as the mid-1990s, aerobic exercise was thought to be the only kind of exercise necessary. Recent research, however, has made it clear that as you age, anaerobic exercise (for example, weight lifting) is equally important.

As in other aspects of exercise, your approach should be dictated by your goals. What do you hope to achieve through weight training? There are many different methods you can apply to weight lifting. To elicit improvements in both muscular strength and endurance, it is best to do eight to twelve repetitions (reps) per set with a moderately heavy weight. A lower rep range of six to eight reps with a heavier weight will better optimize strength and endurance, whereas a lighter weight with fifteen reps will focus more on endurance and toning.

Stretching and a warm-up exercise are equally important with strength training as with cardiovascular training. Doing a warm-up set of an exercise with a light weight will help you retain your form as you move up to heavier weights. Stretching also helps after the workout by lengthening the muscles that you just pumped up.

Savvy weight trainers have developed ways to get the benefits of strength and cardiovascular training from the same activity, effectively cutting their overall workout time in half. Once you have graduated from a novice to a more intermediate or advanced level, you can try lifting weights in a vigorous and uninterrupted fashion, typically at one- to two-minute intervals, to elevate your heart rate almost to the target range. This will provide a combination of anaerobic and aerobic exercise. Another way to combine the two types is to carry hand weights of two to five pounds while walking briskly; this will work your arm muscles and get your heart rate into the target range more quickly.

Expect to experience some muscle soreness after strength training not only right at the beginning, but also each time you increase the weight. Why do you get sore muscles after weight training? Strength training creates small tears in the muscle fibers. The process by which your body repairs these fibers, which takes about forty-eight hours, gives your muscles increased strength. This is why fitness trainers recommend a full day of rest between weight-training sessions. If you lift every day, you will interrupt this mending and strengthening process and will not make progress in steadily increasing your muscle strength.

Weight Machines, Free Weights, and Isometrics

The most popular exercises for upper-body strength training include tricep presses, bicep curls, shoulder presses, lat pull-downs (for strengthening the back), and chest presses. The most popular exercises for lower-body strength training include abdominal crunches, calf raises, leg presses, and leg curls. Most fitness clubs are likely to have multiple machines for each of these popular exercises, and you can also perform these same lifting routines using free weights.

If you would rather avoid pumping iron altogether, you can still get into great shape by using your own body weight to provide resistance. Even if you are a thousand miles away from home and your fitness club, you can maintain your fitness by performing such exercises as push-ups, abdominal crunches, leg lifts, squats, calf raises, and lunges.

Here are some basic strength-training exercises:

1a. Abdominal Curl (Correct)

Contract the abdominal muscles, pulling the ribs toward the pubic bone on the exhale/lift.

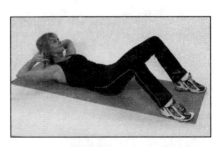

1b. Incorrect Abdominal Curl

Elbows too far forward. Avoid pulling on the neck.

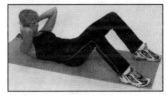

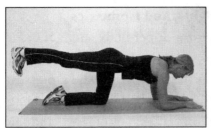

2a. Leg Lift—All-fours position (Correct)

Benefits the buttocks. Gently lift and lower extended leg without lifting above hip height.

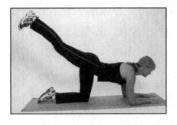

2b. Incorrect Leg Lift

Extended leg is too high. This can stress the lower back.

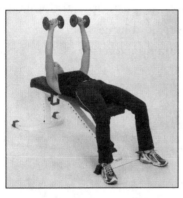

3a. Dumbbell Chest Press— Start Position (Correct)

Benefits the chest, front of the shoulders, and back of the upper arm. Slowly lower weights to chest height.

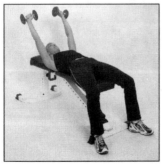

3b. Incorrect Dumbbell Chest Press—Start Position

Weights are too far back. Weights need to be aligned over the chest.

4a. Dumbbell Chest Press— Midpoint (Correct)

Exhale and with a slow controlled movement raise weights back to the start position.

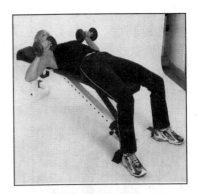

4b. *Incorrect* Dumbbell Chest Press—Midpoint

Weights not in line with the chest; they are too near the shoulders and neck.

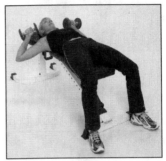

5a. Upright Row (Correct)

An excellent shoulder and upper-back exercise. Lead with the elbows.

5b. *Incorrect* Upright Row

Elbows are too low. Weights are out of alignment.

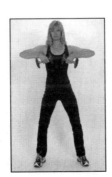

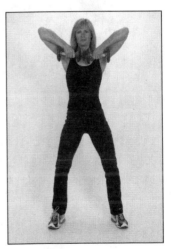

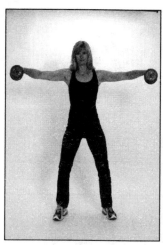

6a. *Lateral Raise (Correct)*
Benefits the shoulders. Elbows slightly flexed, palms facing down. Slowly raise weights to shoulder level.

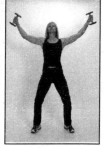

6b. *Incorrect Lateral Raise*
Leaning backward stresses the lower back. Arms are raised far too high.

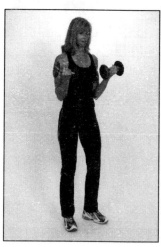

7a. *Biceps Curl (Correct)*
Benefits the muscles of the upper front arm. Stand tall. Keep elbows down and to the sides of the body. Shoulders do not move as the weights are slowly raised and lowered.

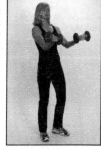

7b. *Incorrect Biceps Curl*
Common errors: arching lower back, throwing elbows forward, moving shoulders.

8a. Standing Triceps Extension (Correct)

Benefits the back of the upper arm. Gently lower weight behind the head on the exhale. Inhale and extend the elbows, lifting the weight above the head.

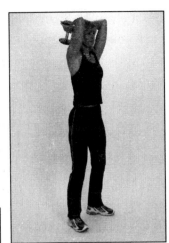

8b. Incorrect Triceps Extension

Avoid leaning backward, arching the lower back. Avoid flaring the elbows out.

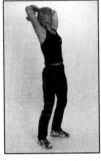

Plateaus and Progress

Your progress in strength training is not unlike the stock market; it cannot go up in a straight line forever. Expect some peaks and an occasional valley and some plateaus in between. Plateaus have long been the nemesis of strength trainers—you get to a certain point, and you do not seem to be making any progress; you cannot add any weight, and in some cases, you cannot lift the same weight or reps that you did a week or two ago. Do not let plateaus erode your confidence and motivation. As long as you avoid overtraining, everything will work out fine; as soon as the plateau is finished, you will have another opportunity to make more progress in your training.

One way to increase the probability of steady progress is to vary your workouts. A personal trainer can also ensure you succeed at this. You can increase your workout challenge and variety in dozens of ways. A few examples include: changing the exercise you do, doing more sets, doing more repetitions per set, adding more weight, shortening intervals of rest between sets, and circuit training (rotating through various types of fitness equipment). Continually making your workouts more challenging helps you power past plateaus and is one way to maximize consistent progress in your training.

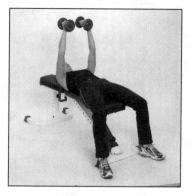

9a. Dumbbell Fly—Start Position (Correct)

Benefits chest and shoulders. Align weights above chest, elbows slightly flexed.

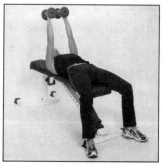

9b. Incorrect Dumbbell Fly— Start Position

Weights are too far back over the face. Elbows are locked.

10a. Dumbbell Fly—Midpoint (Correct)
Lower arms to shoulder height, keeping lower back flat against the bench.

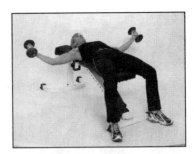

10b. Incorrect Dumbbell Fly—Midpoint
Arms have been lowered below shoulder height.

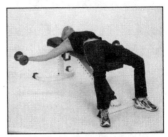

11a. Bent-Over Row— Start Position (Correct)
Benefits the back muscles. Spine should be parallel to the floor.

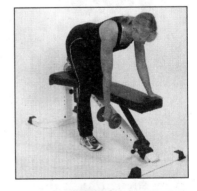

11b. Incorrect Bent-Over Row—Start Position
Back is rounded, abdominals not contracted, working arm is too low.

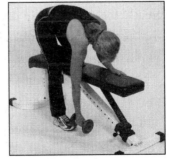

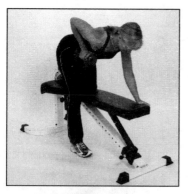

12a. Bent Over Row—
Midpoint (Correct)

Exhale as weight is lifted; keep the working arm close to the body.

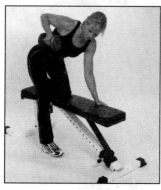

12b. Incorrect Bent-Over
Row—Midpoint

Working arm is raised too high; shoulders are out of alignment.

8. Devote a significant portion of your workout time to flexibility training.

Stretching builds flexibility. You need to stretch following every strength or cardio workout, but you can also benefit greatly from stretching on those days when you do not have another type of workout scheduled. Look into classes in yoga, which is one of the most effective types of flexibility training.

Stretching your muscles in one area should never cause pain in another area of the body. To prevent this kind of pain, stretch slowly and deliberately instead of bouncing up and down or wrenching your limbs abruptly into position. Take your time. Hold each stretch for ten to thirty seconds counting slowing, then release and return slowly to the original position. Bouncing and jerking while stretching can tear your muscles.

Here are some basic stretching exercises that can increase your flexibility in the following target areas:

13a. Hamstring Stretch (Correct)

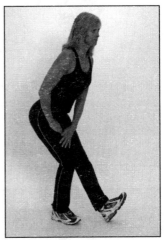

Improves flexibility in the muscles at the back of the legs. Lean forward from the hips, supporting the upper body by placing hands on the thigh.

13b. Incorrect Hamstring Stretch

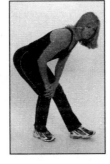

Leaning too far forward. Avoid placing hands on the knee joint.

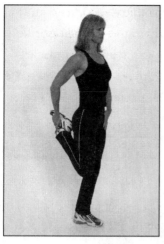

14a. Quadriceps Stretch (Correct)

Stretches the front upper muscles of the leg. Stand tall and contract abdominals, pulling the heel back to the buttocks.

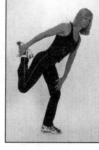

14b. Incorrect Quadriceps Stretch

Leaning too far forward; leg is pulled back too far.

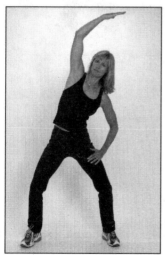

15a. Lateral Stretch (Correct)

Stretches the side of the torso. Support the torso with one hand on the upper thigh, keeping hips squared.

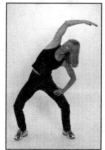

15b. Incorrect Lateral Stretch

Leaning for-ward and too far over to the side; one hip out of alignment can cause ligament damage.

Other simple exercises that promote flexibility include side-to-side looks and ear-to-shoulder stretches for the neck, shoulder shrugs and rolls, and arm circles in which your arms are extended out to the sides at shoulder height.

9. After every workout, cool down and stretch for at least five minutes.

After strength training, stretch out the muscles you just worked to minimize the soreness and stiffness you may experience in the twenty-four to forty-eight hours following your workout. After your cardiovascular training, cool down by doing five minutes of cardio activity at a very low intensity. Do not just stop; you need your heart to return slowly to its normal resting rate.

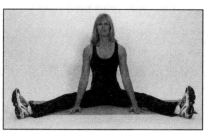

16a. Straddled Stretch (Correct)

Improves flexibility in the back, buttocks, hamstrings, and groin muscles. Sit erect. Pull in abdominals and lean forward from the hips, supporting the torso with the arms extended.

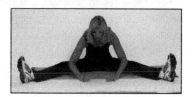

*16b. **Incorrect** Straddle Stretch*

Bending from the waist. Abdominals not contracted; upper torso collapses, stressing the lower back.

10. Vary your routine to keep it fresh and interesting. Keep a log of your exercise plan, activity, and progress.

Motivation is key, which is why this chapter mentions so many ways to increase motivation. Vary the challenge in your workouts by going all out one day and easier than usual the next. Vary the activities you perform; alternate among the swimming pool, rowing machine, and hiking trail on consecutive days. Vary weights, repetitions, sets, and intervals of rest. All these tactics to interject variety into your daily workouts will help keep you on track and help you avoid feeling burned out.

By becoming aware of your favorite excuses not to work out, you can eliminate the obstacles that keep you from getting fit. Exercising first thing in the morning is ideal for many people; you may find that you are less likely to skip a workout because you have to work overtime or are too tired to go to the gym. If you miss workouts because you feel guilty about not spending enough time with the family, bring the family together for a weekend hike or bicycle ride. If being social is your key to consistency, join a group exercise class; take lessons in a sport such as tennis, golf, or racquetball; or find a workout partner and schedule your workouts together weeks in advance.

An exercise log is another tool to keep you motivated. Record the date, what you did, what your goals are for the next workout, and how you felt during and after exercise. Following is an example of an exercise log. You can create a daily, weekly, and monthly log to monitor your activity and progress.

SAMPLE DAILY EXERCISE LOG

DATE: _____

Before working out, I felt: _____

_____

After working out, I felt: _____

_____

TYPE OF EXERCISE

CARDIO	**Time/Reps/Weight**	**Notes/Goals for Next Session**
Treadmill	45 min.	Almost too easy; increase elevation next time to provide more resistance
STRENGTH		
Leg Press	70 lbs.; 3 sets of 12 reps	Felt strong; time to bump weight up to 80 or 90 lbs.
Leg Curl	80 lbs.; 3 sets of 12 reps	Felt looser the last time I did leg curls
FLEXIBILITY		
Stretching	Warm up stretches; stretched quads and hamstrings after workout	Legs pretty tight after workout
Yoga	30 min. class	Instructor really pushed us

Next workout date: _____

Goals for next workout: _____

_____

_____

The exercise log can also help you maximize your workout results and give you the information you need to avoid future injuries. Your log can guide you in pinpointing which types of workouts make you feel good or bad afterward, and which kinds of activities may have contributed to your last injury.

Chapter Summary

A key difference between a youthful person and an elderly one is the disparity in their muscle mass. The benefits of exercise go beyond slowing down the aging process. By adopting a consistent fitness program, you can increase energy and endurance, build strength and flexibility, prevent many diseases, and improve your overall health and vitality. Some studies have even indicated that physical exercise is important for maintaining mental function and memory. Benefits of exercise are linked with proper nutrition and stress management.

Be sure to devote several blocks of time per week to each of the three types of essential exercise: aerobic training, strength training, and flexibility training. Exercise is a healthy outlet and can be a lot of fun. It also improves your attitude and frame of mind. Following the ten recommendations described in this chapter can ensure that you achieve slow and steady progress toward your fitness goals while maximizing optimum health and vitality.

Ten Practical Ways to Commit to an Exercise Program

1. Before beginning your regimen, identify your exercise goals and objectives. To guide you in designing your exercise program and tracking your progress, see a

medical practitioner to obtain a physical exam and base-line medical information.

2. Assess how self-motivated you are. This will determine how you can best maximize the success of your fitness program through the services of a personal trainer, fitness club, or home gym.

3. Work with a certified professional trainer to establish a fitness routine appropriate for your health conditions and fitness objectives.

4. Be consistent with your exercise routine. Work out a minimum of three days per week for at least forty-five minutes.

5. Warm up for at least ten minutes before every workout.

6. Devote a significant portion of your workout time to cardiovascular training.

7. Devote a significant portion of your workout time to strength training.

8. Devote a significant portion of your workout time to flexibility training.

9. After every workout, cool down and stretch for at least five minutes.

10. Vary your routine to keep it fresh and interesting. Keep a log of your exercise plan, activity, and progress.

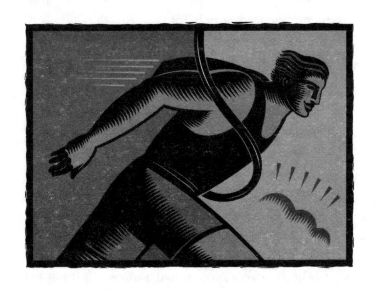

Day by day, step by step, you can make optimum health and vitality a reality.

Summary—Taking Action

If you have taken the time to read and learn from each chapter in this book—congratulations! You are on your way to optimum health and vitality. Living each day with better health and increased vitality is within your reach. It can be realized in a relatively short period of time, depending on your level of commitment and execution.

We don't expect that you will incorporate every recommendation outlined in each chapter immediately; it will be a deliberate process based on your specific health goals and personal motivation. It will be a journey that will require, at times, support from your friends, family members, and various health coaches. We believe the time and energy you dedicate will translate into benefits that are profound and everlasting.

No person can strictly adhere to all the concepts we have described on a daily basis. There are times when it just isn't practical to follow these recommendations. We expect that you will choose your indiscretions with regards to nutrition, stress management, and exercise plans—you are only human. Your daily program may not be as strict when you are on vacation, on a business trip, under tight deadlines, or celebrating a special occasion. That is understandable and acceptable. Our philosophy is "everything in moderation."

You have taken the first step to creating a healthier, more vital, and energetic life just by reading this book. For this you should be proud. You may be feeling, however, a bit over-whelmed at this stage. In fact, you might be asking yourself, "Okay, I have read what to do and how to do it—but where do I start?"

The best place to begin adopting a vitality lifestyle is by cre-ating a personal plan. Before you develop your plan, we suggest that you complete each of the assessments that have been pro-vided within the various chapters. Once completed, utilize a reference source that best allows you to update and refer to your vitality plan: such as a journal—either handwritten or electronic.

In addition to the specific outlines provided for the stress and exercise plans in each of the two chapters, your personal vitality plan might include the following seven sections. Feel free to organize the plan so it works most effectively for you; consider sharing this plan with your support network to solicit their encouragement. Lastly, we suggest that you identify a qualified health practitioner to help guide and monitor your progress throughout this journey.

1. **Assessment scores:** document your scores for each of the assessments for which you have completed.
2. **Health challenges:** document your existing health symp-toms and challenges.
3. **Health goals:** document your health goals, based on your health challenges.
4. **Actions:** document for each, what you plan to do to reach your health goals based on the recommendations provided within this book.

5. **Timeline:** document for each action, the time frame in which you will begin execution. For example, you may choose to begin taking nutritional supplements immediately, and gradually change your dietary habits. Each month thereafter, you can focus on another key vitality factor.

6. **Progress report:** document your progress in each of your goal areas—what challenges you experienced as well as your successes and accomplishments.

7. **Review and update:** be sure to review and update your plan on a regular basis. For some, this will be weekly—for others, it may be monthly or quarterly. Always indicate the date on which you make your comments in your journal.

This book was written based on decades of experience. We have witnessed thousands of people drastically improve their health and vitality. We have succeeded where conventional medicine has failed. This is not a book about fad concepts or marketing hype. It is the essence of our teachings, beliefs, and practices—based on both scientific and empirical research.

The Vitality Connection describes proven and effective techniques you can use and apply today. Other researchers, scientists, and practitioners may refine the principles in this book, but they will not abandon them. These concepts provide the essential core and structure of good health and vitality—which will never go away.

Your task now is to make a commitment to change and grow. By creating your vision of vitality and executing your plan, you can maximize your life. You no longer need to accept the myth that painful aging and poor health is inevitable. You have the possibility of improving your quality of life with optimal health and vitality if you are willing to follow what we recommend. Do not wait—make your commitments now. You are the only one who can make your goals a reality.

May good health and vitality be yours for the rest of your life.

> —Michael J. Grossman, M.D.
> and Jodi L. Jones

Appendix A

Quick Reference Guide

Top Ten Recommendations for Each Key Factor

Key Factor One—Participate in an Anti-Aging Program

Key Factor Two—Develop and Execute a Stress Reduction Plan

Key Factor Three—Create Loving Romantic Relationships

Key Factor Four—Eat Balanced Nutritious Meals

Key Factor Five—Perform a Healthy Kitchen Makeover

Key Factor Six—Supplement Your Diet with Quality Vitamins and Minerals

Key Factor Eight—Conquer Fatigue

If you experience fatigue only on weekdays:

If your fatigue level goes up and down during the day:

Key Factor Nine—Detoxify Your Body

Key Factor Ten—Commit to an Exercise Program

Appendix B
Resources

Anti-Aging / Holistic Health Practitioners
American Academy of Anti-Aging Medicine
2415 N. Greenview
Chicago, IL 60614
1-773-528-8500
www.worldhealth.net

The American College for Advancement in Medicine
23121 Verdugo Drive, Suite 204
Laguna Hills, CA 92653
1-949-583-7666
www.acam.org

American Holistic Health Association
P.O. Box 17400
Anaheim, CA 92817
1-714-779-6152
www.ahha.org

Grossman Wellness and Longevity Medical Center
24432 Muirlands Blvd., Suite 111
Lake Forest, CA 92630
1-949-770-7301
www.ocwellness.com

Wellness Alliance Network, Inc.
111 Pacifica, Suite 250
Irvine, CA 92618
1-949-770-0723
www.wanvitality.com

Cranial Electrotherapy Stimulation

The Alpha-Stim 100 combines microcurrent and cranial electrotherapy stimulator for treatment of pain, anxiety, depression,
insomnia, and related disorders. The Alpha-Stim SCS (Stress Control
System) treats stress-related disorders such as anxiety, depression,
and insomnia. The Alpha-Stim utilizes a small microcurrent stimulator that you clip to your ear lobes for twenty to thirty minutes daily.

Electromedical Products International, Inc.
2201 Garrett Morris Parkway
Mineral Wells, TX 76067
1-800-FOR-PAIN
www.alpha-stim.com

Vitamin MD
P.O. Box 95
River Edge, NJ 07661
1-201-488-4274
www.vitaminmd.com

Facial Rejuvenation Centers

Parisian Peel
Medical Microdermabrasion
1-800-262-4412
www.parisianpeel.com

The Rejuvenation and LaserCare Centers
24432 Muirlands Blvd., Suite 101
Lake Forest, CA 92630
1-949-855-9850
www.ocwellness.com

Financial Planning

The Financial Planning Association
www.fpanet.org

Fitness / Personal Trainers

Aerobics and Fitness Association of America: www.afaa.com
Get Fit: www.getfit.com
International Fitness Association: www.ifafitness.com
Pilates: www.pilates-studio.com
Ultimate One-On-One Personal Training:
    www.UltimatePersonalTraining.com

Nutritious Food Products

Healthy Eating: www.healthy-eating.com
Mother's Market: www.mothersmarket.com
Natural Sugar Substitutes: www.wanvitality.com
Planet Vegan: www.planetvegan.com
The Vegetarian Resource Group: www.vrg.org
Think Organics: www.thinkorganics.com
Trader Joes: www.traderjoes.com
U.S.D.A. Food and Nutrition Information:
    www.nal.usda.gov/fnic
Whole Foods Market: www.wholefoodsmarket.com
USANA Health Sciences: www.usana.com

Healthy Recipes

Cooking Light: www.cookinglight.com
Eating Well: www.eatingwell.com
FoodFit: www.foodfit.com
Nutritiously Gourmet: www.nutritiouslygourmet.com
Vegan Chef: www.veganchef.com
Vegetarian Times: www.vegetariantimes.com
Wellness Alliance Network: www.wanvitality.com

Laboratory Testing Centers

Great Smokies Diagnostic Laboratory
63 Zillicoa Street
Asheville, NC 28801
1-800-522-4762
www.gsdl.com

Doctor's Data, Inc.
301 W. 101 Roosevelt Road
W. Chicago, IL 60185
1-800-323-2784
www.doctorsdata.com

Immunosciences Lab, Inc.
8730 Wilshire Blvd., #305
Beverly Hills, CA 90211
1-800-950-4686
www.immuno-sci-lab.com

Metametrix Clinical Laboratory
5000 Peachtree Industrial Blvd., Suite 110
Nocross, GA 30071
1-800-221-4640
www.metametrix.com

Meditation and Stress Reduction

A taped course in breathing exercises for revitalization is available from Andrew Weil, M.D., at Ask Dr. Weil:
www.drweil.com

The Transcendental Meditation Program is easily learned, extremely beneficial, and has comprehensive follow-up classes:
1-888-532-7686
www.tm.org

One of our favorite practical books on stress reduction is the *Handbook to Higher Consciousness* by Ken Keyes, published in 1972. This book outlines an excellent program for dissolving emotional addictions and blockages to happiness.
www.insightandlove.com

Utilizing gentle, nonintrusive, natural movements, the Trager approach helps release deep-seated physical and mental patterns and facilitates deep relaxation, increased physical mobility, and mental clarity.
Trager International
24800 Chagrin Blvd.
Suite 205
Beachwood, OH 44122
1-216-896-9383
www.Trager.com

Another favorite book is *Love is Letting Go of Fear* by Jerry Jampolsky, M.D., founder of The Center for Attitudinal Healing.
The Center for Attitudinal Healing
33 Buchanan Drive
Sausalito, CA 94965
1-415-331-6161
www.healingcenter.org

Corporate Wellness Team
Chair Massage and Stress Reduction Therapies
www.corporatewellnessteam.com

Nutritional Supplementation

Metagenics
100 Avenida La Pata
San Clemente, CA 92673
1-949-366-0380
www.metagenics.com

NutraNomics, Inc.
11576 South State St.
Suite 1101
Draper, UT 84020
1-800-745-0393
www.nutranomic.com

PhytoPharmica
825 Challenger Drive
Green Bay, WI 54311
1-800-553-2370
www.PhytoPharmica.com

Thorne Research, Inc.
P.O. Box 25
Dover, ID 83825
1-208-263-1337
www.thorne.com

USANA Health Sciences
3838 West Parkway Blvd.
Salt Lake City, UT 84120
1-888-950-9595
www.usana.com

Vitamin MD
P.O. Box 95
River Edge, NJ 07661
1-201-488-4274
www.vitaminmd.com

Physiological Aging Testing Practitioners
ActualAge Directory: www.wellnesswatchers.com

Relationship Enrichment
Barbara R. Grossman, Ph.D.
Individual, Marriage and Family Counseling
24432 Muirlands Blvd., Suite 111
Lake Forest, CA 92630
1-949-230-1429
www.ocwellness.com

National Marriage Encounter
1-800-828-3351
www.marriage-encounter.org
The above resource is for marriage enrichment; it is not intended for couples in crisis.

Imago Relationship Therapy
1-800-729-1121
www.imagotherapy.com

Skin Care
Aesthetic Technologies
1-800-262-4412
www.parisianpeel.com

Sense' Beautiful Science, USANA Health Sciences
1-888-950-9595
www.usana.com

N.V. Perricone, M.D. Cosmeceuticals
1-203-379-0726
www.clinicalcreations.com

The Rejuvenation and LaserCare Centers
1-949-855-9850
www.ocwellness.com

Wellness Education and Vitality Workshops

Wellness Alliance Network, Inc.
111 Pacifica, Suite 250
Irvine, CA 92618
1-949-770-0723
www.wanvitality.com

Appendix C
Glycemic Index Chart

The glycemic index (GI) was first developed by Davis Jenkins in 1981. It is a numerical system of measuring how fast a carbohydrate triggers a rise in circulating blood sugar—the higher the number, the greater the blood sugar response. A low GI food will cause a small rise, while a high GI food will trigger a dramatic spike. A list of common carbohydrates with their glycemic values is shown below. We have listed, by category, those with higher GI numbers in descending values (highest to lowest).

The glycemic index is used as a guideline for dietary recommendations for people with either diabetes or hypoglycemia. Individuals with blood sugar problems are advised to avoid foods with high values and should instead choose carbohydrate-containing foods with lower values. The glycemic index should not be the only dietary guideline. We recommend that you also consider other nutritional values such as fat, protein, fiber, cholesterol, and sodium.

COMMON FOODS	GLYCEMIC INDEX
Sugars	
Maltose	105
Glucose	100
Sucrose	83

Honey	75
Fructose	20
Xylitol	7

Fruits

Raisins	64
Bananas	62
Papaya	60
Orange juice	46
Grapes	45
Strawberries	40
Oranges	40
Apples	39
Tomatoes	38
Pears	34
Grapefruit	26
Peaches	26
Plums	25
Cherries	24

Vegetables

French fries	107
Potato, baked	98
Parsnips	97
Potato (new), boiled	70
Beets	64
Sweet potato	51
Green peas	51
Carrot, cooked	36
Carrot, raw	31

Grains

Puffed rice	95
Cornflakes	80
Whole-grain wheat bread	72
White rice	70
White bread	69
Wheat cereal	67
Corn	59
Brown rice	55
Bran cereal	51
White spaghetti	50
Oatmeal	49
Pasta	45
Whole-grain rye bread	42
Whole-wheat spaghetti	42

Legumes and Nuts

Chick peas	39
Lima beans	36
Lentils	29
Kidney beans	29
Soybeans	15
Nuts	13

Appendix D
Nutritional Recommendations

Nutritional Supplementation

In addition to the benefits described in Chapter Six, nutritional supplementation becomes even more critical as we get older. However, people of all age groups and health conditions can benefit. As we age, we lose our ability to manufacture certain enzymes and nutrients; we also lose the ability to effectively absorb nutrients from the foods we eat. The natural aging process requires higher doses of vitamins and minerals to protect us from the effects of aging.

Based on the criteria outlined in Chapter Six, we recommend you take quality nutritional supplements that meet the following guidelines:

1. The supplements should be scientifically formulated and balanced with the proper ratio of nutrients.
2. The manufacturer should follow Good Manufacturing Practices (GMP) and comply with U.S. Pharmacological (USP) Standards for pharmaceutical-grade products.
3. The products should be independently tested and guaranteed for potency and safety.
4. The products should be manufactured by a reputable company that maintains scientific research and development.

5. The products should be recommended by nutrition-oriented health practitioners and listed in the the Physician's Desk Reference.
6. The trace minerals should be chelated and provided in their most bioavailable (absorbable) form.

OPTIMAL INTAKE RANGE FOR VITAMINS AND MINERALS

Vitamins	Range for Adults
Vitamin A (retinol)	5,000 IU[1]
Vitamin A (from beta-carotene and mixed carotenoids)	5,000–25,000 IU
Vitamin D	100–400 IU
Vitamin E (d-alpha tocopherol, gamma and delta tocopherol)	100v800 IU
Vitamin K (phytonadione)	60–100 mcg
Vitamin C (ascorbic acid)	100–1,000 mg
Bioflavanoid complex	100–200 mg
Vitamin B_1 (thiamin)	10–100 mg
Vitamin B_2 (riboflavin)	10v50 mg
Niacin	10–100mg
Niacinamide	10–30 mg
Vitamin B_6 (pyridoxine)	25–100 mg
Biotin	100–300 mcg
Pantothenic acid	25–100 mg
Folic acid	400–800 mcg
Vitamin B_{12}	400–1,000 mcg
Choline	10–100 mg
Inositol	10–100 mg

Minerals

Calcium	750–1,500 mg [2]
Chromium	200–400 mcg [3]
Copper	1–3 mg
Iodine	150–225 mcg
Iron	10–30 mg [4]
Magnesium	300–750 mg
Manganese	1–5 mg
Molybdenum	10–100 mcg
Selenium	100–200 mcg
Vanadium	30–50 mcg
Zinc	15–30 mg

Optional

Silica	1–25 mg
Boron	1–6 mg

Phytonutrients

Various phytonutrients such as tumeric, lutein, broccoli, quercetin, alpha-carotene, bilberry, and lycopene.

1. Women of childbearing age should take not take more than 2,500 IU of retinol daily if becoming pregnant is a possibility, due to the risk of birth defects.
2. Taking a separate calcium supplement may be necessary in women at risk or suffering from osteoporosis.
3. For diabetes and weight loss, dosages of 600 mcg can be used.
4. For menstruating women only. Men and postmenopausal women rarely need supplemental iron.

Nutritional Supplementation Recommendations

At a minimum, the average adult should take the following nutritional supplements. For maximum absorption and to reduce any potential stomach upset, we recommend you take your nutritional supplements with food. Most people tolerate their nutritional program without any problems.

Multivitamins
Dosage Recommendations
See optimal intake ranges in preceding table.

Omega 3 Fish Oil
Dosage Recommendations
1000 mcg twice daily.

CoEnzyme Q10 (CoQ10)
Dosage Recommendations
30 mg twice daily (after age forty).

Calcium
Dosage Recommendations
300–600 mg twice daily.

Vitamin E with Mixed Alpha, Gamma and Delta Tocopherols
Dosage Recommendations
200 IU: Take 1 tablet twice daily.

Grape Seed Extract (Proanthocyanidins)
Dosage Recommendations
30–100 mg once daily.

Additional Supplementation Recommendations Based on Specific Health Conditions

In addition to the nutritional products listed previously, below is a brief summary of additional recommendations for those with specific health conditions. These recommendations are not comprehensive and do not include diet or exercise recommendations. You should consult a medical practitioner before treating an illness with nutritional supplements, changing your diet, or beginning an exercise regimen.

Anti-aging Hormonal Recommendations

Obtain a blood test to measure Free T-3 and Free T-4 levels; if abnormal consider natural thyroid supplementation.

Men over 40

- Take 25–50 mg of DHEA and check blood levels for DHEA absorption.
- Use testosterone cream and check blood levels for absorption.

Women over 40

- Take 15–25 mg of DHEA and check blood levels for DHEA absorption.
- Use small doses of testosterone cream.

Men and Women over 40

- Growth Hormone Releasing Factor: Take 5 days per week.
- Melatonin: Take 0.5 to 1 mg at bedtime.

Arthritis / Joint Pain (including Lupus)
Dosage Recommendations
- Glucosamine sulfate: 500 mg three times daily or 1,000 mg twice daily (it will take six weeks to produce results).
- MSM (methylsulfonomethane-organic sulfur): 2,000–3,000 mg twice daily.
- DHEA: 25 mg for women and 50 mg for men per day taken in morning.
- Pancreatin: 350–750 mg between meals, three times daily, or bromelain: 250–750 mg (1,800 to 2,000 mcu) between meals three times daily.
- L-glutamine: 1 gram, two to three times daily to heal intestinal lining.
- N-Acetylcysteine: 100–250 mg once daily.

Botanical Recommendations
- Boswellia extract: 400–800 mg, three times daily.
- Tumeric extract: 300–600 mg, three times daily.
- Ginger extract: 200–400 mg, three times daily.
- Quercetin: 100–200 mg, three times daily.

Cardiovascular Disease: Atherosclerosis and Heart Disease

Cardiovascular disease is responsible for at least 43 percent of all deaths in the United States. Atherosclerosis, the process of hardening of the arteries, can be stopped and even reversed through dietary and lifestyle change. Type A behavior and worrying are linked to heart disease. Cigarette smoke should be strictly avoided. Reduced antioxidant levels have been shown to be as important, or possibly more important, than high cholesterol in predicting a person's likelihood of having a stroke or heart attack.

Vitamin E supplementation has been shown to significantly reduce the risk of heart attack. Take vitamin E as mixed tocopherols 200 mg twice daily.

General prevention for cardiovascular disease must include 1,000 mg of fish oil twice daily. Fish oil is the single most effective supplement to help reduce the risk of heart attacks and strokes.

In many cases, EECP (enhanced external counterpulsation) or EDTA chelation therapy is a suitable alternative to coronary angioplasty or bypass surgery.

Atherosclerosis: Hardening of the Arteries

Artherosclerosis is detected by CardioVision as an arterial stiffness index, and can be treated effectively with PlaqueOff, an herbal combination with oral EDTA. Take one or two tablets three times daily. Improvement can be measured in four to eight weeks and should continue as long as you remain on a quality supplement program.

Reducing the risk of heart disease and strokes involves eliminating as many risk factors as possible. Consult your physician regarding blood tests for homocysteine, lipoprotein(a), fibrinogen, and C-reactive protein; abnormal results will require treatment of the condition. New blood tests for advanced detection of fractionated lipid profile are available from Great Smokies Laboratory: total and fractionated VLDL, and fractionated HDL and LDL density pattern can be tested and treated.

Heart Disease: Congestive Heart Failure, Arrhythmia, Mitral Valve Prolapse, and Cardiomyopathy

Dosage Recommendations

- Vitamin C: 500 mg three times daily.
- Vitamin E (mixed tocopherols): 800 IU once daily.
- Fish oil: 1,000 mg twice daily *or* Flaxseed oil: 1 tablespoon once daily.
- Magnesium: 200–400 mg three times daily.
- Coenzyme Q10: 100 mg twice daily.
- L-Carnitine: 300 mg three times daily.
- Taurine: 500–600 mg 1 tablet, twice daily.
- Hawthorne extract: 300–600 mg 1 tablet, three times daily.

Chronic Fatigue Syndrome

Refer to the chapters on Balancing Your Immune System, Detoxifying Your Body, and Conquering Fatigue.

Depression

Dosage Recommendations

- Flaxseed oil or fish oil: Take 1,000 mg twice daily or one tablespoon daily.
- SAMe: Take 200 mg twice daily; you should see results in five days.
- 5-HTTP: Take 100–200 mg three times daily; you should see results in two to three weeks.
- Folic acid: Take 2 mg twice daily.

If depression has not improved in three weeks, add St. John's wort extract 300 mg three times daily.

If anxiety is a significant factor, take 45–70 mg kavalactones (standardized kava extract) three times daily.

Diabetes
Dosage Recommendations
- Bitter gourd extract (Momordica charantia): 150–300 mg, twice daily.
- Gymnema extract: 100mg–200 mg, twice daily.
- Alpha lipoic acid: 100–300 mg, twice daily.
- Vanadyl sulfate: 3–5 mg, twice daily.
- Chromium: 300 mcg 2, twice daily.

Exercise is critical. Follow an exercise program that elevates your heart rate to at least 60 percent of your target heart rate for one-half hour, five to six times per week. Refer to the exercise chapter in this book.

Diet
All simple processed and concentrated carbohydrates must be avoided; the consumption of complex carbohydrate, high-fiber foods, including legumes, should be consumed. Alcohol consumption must be avoided.

Elevated Homocysteine Levels
Dosage Recommendations
- Vitamin B_6: 25–50 mg once daily.
- Vitamin B_{12} (Methylcobalamine): 1,000–2,000 mg once daily; sublingual formula (under the tongue for better absorption).

- Folic acid: 400–800 mcg twice daily.
- Trimethyglycine: 500–2,000 mg once daily.

If homocysteine level is not at 10 or below within six weeks, change folic acid to 5-formyl tetrahydrafolate, which is required by some people who have a genetic variation.

Fibromyalgia

Refer to the chapters on Balancing Your Immune System, Detoxifying Your Body, and Conquering Fatigue.

High Cholesterol and Low HDL
Dosage Recommendations

- Niacin as hexaniacinate: Take 500–1,000 mg two or three times daily. (It is important to get a blood test to monitor your liver enzymes two months after starting niacin.)
- Gugulipid (Aryuvedic herb): Take 500 mg once daily.
- Cholessen-red yeast extract: Take 500 mg twice daily.
- Policosanol: Bees wax product: Take 10–20 mg once daily.

Take any or all the above and have your doctor check your cholesterol blood tests. Improvement should occur within six weeks of taking the above recommendations.

Hypoglycemia and Insulin Resistance

Elevated insulin levels can be measured on fasting blood tests and two hours after eating. In addition, a blood test called C'peptide can be taken as a single fasting measurement of insulin levels. If you have diabetes, your glucose level will already be elevated. If your insulin levels or C'peptide are high, you are considered to be prediabetic.

The primary treatment of hypoglycemia is the use of dietary therapy to stabilize blood sugar levels. Diabetes is a complex set of symptoms caused by faulty carbohydrate metabolism induced by a diet too high in refined carbohydrates.

Diet

All simple processed and concentrated carbohydrates must be avoided; the consumption of complex carbohydrate, high-fiber foods, including legumes, should be consumed. Alcohol consumption must be avoided as it can cause hypoglycemia. Frequent small meals with protein stabilize blood sugar levels. Use pure protein powder with one or two scoops in V-8 juice or other low-sugar beverages, such as unsweetened soy milk. Add a scoop of a natural fiber concentrate.

Dosage Recommendations

- Vitamin B_5 (pantothenic acid): 500 mg twice daily.
- Bioflavanoids: 100 mg twice daily.
- Vitamin B_6: 100 mg twice daily.
- Licorice root extract: 300 mg, one to three tablets twice daily.
- Ashwagandha root extract: 50 mg, one to three tablets twice daily.

If you do not feel better within three weeks, add an adrenal gland extract and follow the manufacturer's recommended starting dose.

If you do not feel significantly better within an additional three weeks, increase dosage to the maximum recommendations of the manufacturer.

Irritable Bowel Syndrome

Follow the suggestions outlined in the Stress Reduction and Immune System chapters.

Dosage Recommendations

- Take a rice-based protein powder to decrease likelihood of allergic reactions.
- Follow the instructions for the Elimination Diet in Appendix F.
- Take a good bacterial probiotic with at least 6 billion acidophilus and bifodophilus twice daily.
- Take psyllium husks (natural fiber): one teaspoon once or twice per day to keep stools soft.

Macular Degeneration and Other Eye Diseases

Dosage Recommendations

- Grape seed extract: 30–100 mg once daily.
- Lutein: 5 mg once daily.
- Bilberry: 30 mg once daily.
- Vitamin C: 1000 mg twice daily.
- Vitamin E: 200 mg mixed tocopherols once daily.
- Selenium: 200 mcg once daily.

Memory Loss

Dosage Recommendations

- Acetyl L Carnitine: 200–500 mg, twice daily.

- Ginkgo extract: 40–80 mg, two to three times daily.
- Phosphatidylserine: 100 mg, two to three times daily.
- NADH: 5 mg, once daily in the morning with no food for one hour.

Menopause

Many natural measures can help alleviate the most common symptoms of menopause. The latest research as of 2002 shows an increase in breast and uterine cancer from using Premarin (Horse mare urine estrogens) and Provera (synthetic progestins called methoxyprogesterone). Natural progesterone (identical to human progesterone) combined with human estrogen as estradiol and estriol has been shown to reduce cancer incidence.

Dosage Recommendations
- Black Cohosh: 100–200 mg, twice daily.
- Chasteberry: 100 mg, twice daily.

Diet

Increase the amount of phytoestrogens in the diet by consuming more soy foods, fennel, celery, parsley, high-lignan organic flaxseed oil, nuts, and seeds.

For more intense hormonal support use Estriol or Estradiol-natural progesterone. Cream and sublingual forms are best because they do not need to be processed through the liver. A compounding pharmacist can create any combination your medical doctor prescribes. Usually a biestrogen of Estriol and Estradiol with progesterone as a cream or tablet is recommended. When using these natural hormones, you may need to start at lower doses in the first weeks to reduce the temporary effect of breast tenderness.

Migraine Headache

Following the elimination diet program described in Appendix F is critical. Food is often the primary factor with those suffering from migraine headaches.

Premenstrual Syndrome (PMS)

If you have premenstrual cramps, irritability, or breast tenderness:

- Use natural progesterone cream providing 50 mg of progesterone, once or twice daily.
- Primrose oil: 500–1,000 mg, twice daily.
  or
- Borage oil providing 150–250 mg of GLA, twice daily.

Diet

Eliminate sugar intake; increase your intake of soy foods; eliminate caffeine intake; and keep salt intake low.

Prostate Enlargement

Dosage Recommendations

- Zinc: 45–60 mg once daily.
- Lycopene: 10 mg once daily.

Botanical Recommendations

- Saw palmetto extract (standardized to contain 85 to 95 percent fatty acids and sterols): 160 mg twice daily.
- Flower pollen extract (e.g., Prostat brand): Take one to two tabs twice daily.

- Pygeum Africanum extract (standardized to contain 14 percent triterpenes including beta-sitosterol and 0.5 percent n-docosanol): Take 50–100 mg twice daily.
- Stinging nettle extract: Take 300–600 mg once daily.

Stress
Dosage Recommendations
- Cordyceps mycelium extract: 400 mg once daily.
- Asian ginseng root extract: 200 mg once daily.
- Rhodiola root extract: 50 mg once daily.

Toxicity
See Appendix F for specific recommendations on detoxification. Also, read Chapter Eight on detoxifying your body.

Appendix E
Top Ten Recipes for Vitality

The following offers a variety of delectable options for creating balanced nutritious meals. These are the top ten vitality recipes that we have tested and shared with hundreds of individuals who have attended our Taste of Vitality cooking classes over the past couple of years. Even those who are strict "meat and potatoes people" have made these recipes part of their regular diet. We encourage you to try each recipe and judge for yourself. We are confident that your journey to better health and vitality through healthy cooking will be both rewarding and pleasurable. Bon appétit.

—Jodi L. Jones and
Sally Foster Schneider

Recommend meal key:

B	=	Breakfast
L	=	Lunch
S	=	Snack
D	=	Dinner
Des =		Dessert

Please note: As appropriate, the ingredients listed within the following recipes assume organic fruits and vegetables, as well as non-GMO (genetically modified) soy products.

Top Ten Vitality Recipes

1. Oh So Good Oats (B)
2. Granola Mania (B/L/S/Des)
3. Vitality Boosting Smoothie (B/L/S)
4. Veggie Plus Frittata (B/L/D)
5. Tropical Couscous with Shrimp (L/D)
6. Brown Rice and Vegetable Salad (L/D)
7. Grilled Salmon with Lemon Mint Sauce (L/D)
8. Very Veggie Stuffed Peppers (L/D)
9. Citrus Spinach Salad with Chicken (L/D)
10. Banana Berry Sundae (Des)

1. Oh So Good Oats

This is a traditional oatmeal dish made tasty. Quick or instant oatmeal has virtually no nutritional value and is primarily loaded with simple carbohydrates. This recipe gives you a great way to start your day the "old fashion" way.

Serves: 2–4

Ingredients

1 cup apple juice or apple cider
1 cup filtered water
1 tablespoon cinnamon
1 cup steel-cut oats
2 tablespoons walnut pieces
2 tablespoons sunflower seeds
1 banana

Directions

Bring juice, water, and cinnamon to a boil in a saucepan. Stir in oats and boil over medium heat for 5 minutes. Turn off heat and keep covered for 30 minutes. Oats will be slightly crunchy and all the water should be absorbed into the oats. You do not want to overcook the oats as they will lose their nutritional value. Stir in walnuts and sunflower seeds, warm mixture over low heat for 5 minutes. Add sliced banana (or any other fruit of your choice). Spoon into bowls and serve immediately.

Nutritional Value Per Serving
Calories: 395
Total fat: 11 g
Saturated fat: <1 g
Protein: 20 g
Carbohydrate: 54 g
Sodium: 112 mg
% Fat: 25
% Protein: 20
% Carbohydrates: 55

2. **Granola Mania**
Who says granola has to be boring? With this recipe, you can enjoy granola for breakfast, lunch, snack, or a light dinner. Kids and adults alike give it a "ten" rating! It's simple, quick, and filling.
Serves: 4

Ingredients
6 ounces cultured soy (nondairy yogurt)—flavor of choice
6 ounces organic vanilla yogurt

4 cups natural low-sugar, low-fat granola cereal

1 cup fresh berries (blueberries, raspberries, or straw-berries)

$^1/_2$ cup chopped walnuts

Directions

Combine soy and yogurt and stir until smooth. Spoon equal amounts of the soy-yogurt mixture into four individual bowls. Top the mixture with granola, berries, and walnuts with desired amounts and serve.

Nutritional Value Per Serving

Calories: 380

Total fat: 9 g

Saturated fat: 0 g

Protein: 30 g

Carbohydrate: 51 g

Sodium: 256 mg

% Fat: 20

% Protein: 30

% Carbohydrates: 50

3. Vitality Boosting Smoothie

Ideal for breakfast, lunch, or snack, this recipe includes an ideal balance of protein, carbohydrates, fiber, and essential fatty acids to sustain your energy. You've never tasted a protein smoothie with so much zest, and without the chalky taste of protein powder.

Serves: 1 (main meal) or 2 (snacks)

Ingredients:

1 cup nonfat vanilla soymilk

$^3/_4$ cup frozen mixed berries (or frozen fruit of choice)

$^1/_2$ medium banana (place other half in plastic bag
and refrigerate, eat within 48 hours)
1 tablespoon essential fatty acids
1 tablespoon protein powder
1 tablespoon low-sugar fiber powder

Directions

Using a high-powered blender, combine the soymilk,
frozen berries, and banana. Once fully blended, add
the essential fatty acids, protein powder, and fiber
powder. Blend for thirty seconds until well combined.
Pour into a tall glass with a straw and enjoy.

*For a lower carbohydrate and reduced-calorie ver-
sion, eliminate the banana and/or the soy milk
(replace with water). In addition to the frozen fruit,
add ice to thicken to preference.*

Nutritional Value Per Serving

Calories: 302
Total fat: 6 g
Saturated fat: 0 g
Protein: 28 g
Carbohydrate: 36 g
Sodium: 372 mg
% Fat: 20
% Protein: 35
% Carbohydrates: 45

4. Veggie Plus Frittata

This dish satisfies the appetite of all types, even for the meaty omelet lovers. It is scrumptious just as it stands; if you have a craving for something more substantial, try adding a few tablespoons of soy ground "beef" or chopped soy "ham." You won't believe the flavor enveloping this "egg casserole" based primarily on egg whites and nutrient-rich vegetables. It can be prepared and cooked a day in advance and heated the following day for breakfast, lunch, or dinner.

Serves: 4

Ingredients

Frittata

1 tablespoon extra-virgin olive oil

2 tablespoons shallot, peeled and diced

6 ounces sliced button mushrooms

2 cups spinach, stemmed, washed, and chopped

7 egg whites (if using fresh eggs, whisk egg whites until slightly frothy; otherwise use prepared egg whites)

1 free-range, omega-3 fortified egg

$\frac{1}{4}$ cup low-fat cheese or spicy tofu–rella cheese, grated

Zest of one lemon

3 dashes of hot pepper sauce

1 large Roma tomato, cored and diced

$\frac{1}{4}$ teaspoon dried oregano

$\frac{1}{4}$ teaspoon dried dill weed

Salt and cracked black pepper to taste

Chunky tomato sauce

2 cloves garlic, peeled and sliced
1 large Roma tomato, cored and diced
1 teaspoon extra-virgin olive oil
Dash cayenne pepper
Salt and cracked black pepper to taste

Directions

Preheat oven to 300 degrees.

Chunky Tomato Sauce

Heat a small saucepan with olive oil. Add garlic and cook until golden brown in color. Add tomatoes and cayenne pepper and stew over medium heat for about 10 minutes. The tomatoes will break down and the sauce will become thick and chunky. Season with salt and pepper and keep warm. Stir in a tablespoon of water if the sauce becomes too thick.

Frittata

Chop the prewashed spinach in food processor or by hand. Heat a 10-inch non-stick sauté pan. Add olive oil and diced shallot. Sauté shallots until clear and add sliced mushrooms. Sauté mushrooms until half way cooked and add spinach. Season vegetables with oregano, dill, pepper, and salt; sauté for another 30 seconds, allowing the spinach to wilt.

In a medium bowl, stir egg whites, egg, pepper sauce, oregano, dill, lemon zest, salt, and pepper until well combined. Pour mixture over vegetable sauté to ensure ample coverage of vegetables. Add diced tomatoes. Top with cheese or tofu-rella nondairy cheese.

Cover and cook over low heat for 10 minutes. Transfer sauté pan to preheated oven and heat for 15 minutes, or until egg whites are completely cooked and set. You may need to place this dish under the broiler for a few minutes to set and lightly brown the top (keep an eye on this, you don't want to burn or over cook your frittata). Remove baked frittata from oven and let set for 5 minutes. Cut into 4 equal wedges and serve with a dollop of the fresh chunky tomato sauce. Garnish with fresh fruit and serve.

Nutritional Value Per Serving

Calories: 117
Total fat: 3 g
Saturated fat: 0 g
Protein: 11 g
Carbohydrate: 10 g
Sodium: 201 mg
% Fat: 29
% Protein: 37
% Carbohydrates: 34

5. Tropical Couscous with Shrimp

This colorful, texture-rich dish works as well warm as it does cold. The pineapple juice adds a nice tang and sweetness. Try varying the recipe with dried cherries or dried apricots instead of the raisins. If you have time, lightly toast the almonds in a dry skillet or in the oven. Cilantro also tastes great in place of the mint. Shrimp can be simmered in juice, sautéed, grilled, or broiled; however you prefer to cook them.

Serves: 6

Ingredients

> 30 medium-size raw shrimp, thawed if frozen (not quite 2 pounds)
>
> 3 cups pineapple juice
>
> 2 cups whole-wheat couscous
>
> $1/4$ cup fresh mint leaves, chopped
>
> $1/3$ cup chopped green onion
>
> $1/4$ cup golden raisins or a raisin medley
>
> $1/4$ cup sliced almonds
>
> Salt and fresh ground black pepper to taste

Directions

Clean and devein shrimp. In a sauté pan bring 1 cup of pineapple juice to a simmer over medium heat. Place shrimp in a single layer in the sauté pan and simmer until bright pink; turn once, a few minutes per side, until tender and done. Season to taste with salt and pepper.

As the shrimp are simmering, bring 2 cups of pineapple juice to a boil in a covered medium saucepan. Add couscous and stir. Remove from heat. Allow it to sit, covered, for 5 minutes. Fluff with a fork. Stir in mint, green onion, raisins, and almonds. Season with salt and fresh ground pepper to taste. Arrange couscous on a platter and top with the shrimp. Garnish with extra green onion and mint.

Nutritional Value Per Serving
   Calories: 117
   Total fat: 3 g
   Saturated fat: 0 g
   Protein: 11 g
   Carbohydrate: 10 g
   Sodium: 483 mg
   % Fat: 29
   % Protein: 37
   % Carbohydrates: 34

6. Brown Rice and Vegetable Salad

Recipe adapted from: www.foodfit.com
Serves: 4

Ingredients
   1 cup cooked brown rice (see recipe in The Basics
      section of this appendix)
   1 medium zucchini
   2 stalks celery
   1 carrot
   1 yellow bell pepper
   $\frac{1}{2}$ bunch arugula
   4 scallions
   2 tablespoons fresh lemon juice
   $\frac{1}{4}$ cup chicken or vegetable stock
   1 tablespoon coarse-grained mustard
   1 tablespoon olive oil
   $\frac{1}{2}$ teaspoon salt
   $\frac{1}{4}$ teaspoon fresh ground black pepper

Directions

Cut the zucchini, celery, carrot, and bell pepper into ³/₄-inch dice. Remove the tough stems from the arugula and chop the leaves. Chop the scallions. Blanch the zucchini, celery, carrot and bell pepper for 1 minute. Drain in a colander and immerse in ice water. Drain the vegetables well. In a large bowl, whisk together the lemon juice, stock, mustard, oil, salt, and pepper. Add the rice, blanched vegetables, arugula, and scallions and toss well to combine. Adjust the salt and pepper to taste and serve at room temperature.

Nutritional Value Per Serving

Calories: 168
Total fat: 4 g
Saturated fat: 1 g
Protein: 5 g
Carbohydrate: 19 g
Sodium: 396 mg
% Fat: 23
% Protein: 11
% Carbohydrates: 66

7. Poached Salmon with Lemon Mint Sauce

This dish is just as appetizing warm or chilled. We recommend eating salmon, together with fresh organic leafy greens, at least two times a week (preferably three). Whether following this recipe, or another healthful one, salmon is beneficial to your health. No other fish offers an abundance of protein and essential fatty acids such as fresh, organic, farm-raised salmon. Purchase the freshest salmon and prepare it the same day if possible.

Serves: 4

Ingredients

Lemon Mint Sauce

1 cup plain nonfat yogurt (or half yogurt and half
    nonfat sour cream)
Juice of one-half lemon
$\frac{1}{2}$ teaspoon lemon zest
1 teaspoon dried mint (or 1 tablespoon fresh mint
    leaves, chopped)
Salt and white pepper to taste

Poached Salmon

Juice of 2 lemons
$\frac{1}{2}$ teaspoon seafood seasoning
4 fresh salmon fillets, 5 ounces each
1 cucumber, peeled, halved, and seeded

Directions

Lemon Mint Sauce

Combine all ingredients in a small bowl. Cover and refrigerate for one hour before serving. Can be made up to two days in advance.

Yields: 1 cup

Poached Salmon

Place the lemon juice, salt, seasoning, and 2 cups of water in a 10-inch saucepan. Add the (rinsed) salmon fillets and more water to cover the salmon if necessary.

Bring the liquid to a simmer over medium heat. Remove the fillets when they are just opaque, about 4 minutes depending on thickness. Place the fillets in the refrigerator to cool, or if you prefer warm poached salmon, cover and keep warm. If opting for chilled salmon, you can poach it in advance and keep it covered in the refrigerator for up to 2 days.

Thinly slice the cucumber and divide the slices between 4 plates. Place each chilled salmon fillet on top of the sliced cucumbers. Drizzle the sauce on the salmon and around the plate. Garnish with mint leaves and lemon wedges if desired.

Nutritional Value Per Serving

Calories: 335

Total fat: 4 g

Saturated fat: 0 g

Protein: 36 g

Carbohydrate: 38 g

Sodium: 108 mg

% Fat: 12

% Protein: 43

% Carbohydrates: 45

8. Very Veggie Stuffed Peppers

From stuffed cabbage to stuffed mushrooms, no other stuffed vegetable tastes so rich, sweet, and satisfying. These peppers are so tasty you won't believe how healthy they truly are. Serve as a main course with a green leafy salad, or serve a half portion as a side dish to grilled halibut or salmon (as a source for additional protein). Save time by preparing this dish a day in advance and warming for your planned meal.

Serves: 4–6

Ingredients

> 4 medium sweet red peppers (or bell pepper of choice)
>
> 6 ounces garbanzo beans
>
> ¼ cup walnuts
>
> 1 cup button mushrooms (4 ounces)
>
> ¾ cup cooked brown basmati rice (see in The Basics section of this appendix)
>
> ½ cup soy ground "beef" (taco version adds a lot of flavor)
>
> ¼ cup sunflower seeds
>
> 2 cups organic spaghetti sauce
>
> ¼ cup low-fat mozzarella cheese
>
> 2 tablespoons Parmesan cheese

Directions

Preheat oven to 350 degrees.

Rinse and drain garbanzo beans. Cut bell peppers in half lengthwise, remove seeds, and trim excess membranes. Rinse and pat dry. In a food processor, coarsely chop the walnuts; add garbanzo beans and mushrooms and continue to coarsely chop. In a large bowl, combine chopped walnuts, garbanzo beans, mushrooms, sunflower seeds, brown rice, soy ground "beef," 1 cup of organic marinara sauce, and mozzarella cheese. Salt and pepper to taste. Mix well.

Spoon mixture generously into pepper halves. Sprinkle a small amount of Parmesan cheese over top.

Place stuffed peppers into glass baking dish. Add enough water to lightly cover the bottom of the dish. Cover with foil. Bake in preheated oven for 35 minutes. Remove foil and bake another 10 minutes.

Heat remaining 1 cup of the marinara sauce; add choice of spices if desired (oregano, cayenne pepper, and/or parsley). Arrange peppers halves on platter and serve with heated marinara sauce.

Nutritional Value Per Serving

Calories: 201
Total fat: 10 g
Saturated fat: 1 g
Protein: 12 g
Carbohydrate: 44 g
Sodium: 407 mg
% Fat: 29
% Protein: 16
% Carbohydrates: 55

9. Citrus Spinach Salad with Chicken

There is nothing more refreshing than a crisp green salad tossed with a variety of fresh ingredients. Add a citrus zest and fresh chicken breast, and you've got a complete satisfying meal. Be creative by adding your own selection of vegetables to make this hearty salad your own creation.
Serves: 4

Ingredients

Salad

8 ounces organic baby spinach

1 medium red bell pepper, thinly sliced

12 fresh asparagus spears

6 ounces sliced mushrooms

$3/4$ cup dried cranberries or raisins

6 ounces mandarin oranges, drained

2 tablespoons sliced almonds

4 cooked boneless, skinless chicken breasts (see in The Basics section of this Appendix)

Feta or goat cheese (optional)

Dressing

$1/4$ cup extra-virgin olive oil

1 teaspoon balsamic vinegar

$1/4$ cup orange juice (preferably fresh squeezed)

zest of $1/2$ orange

Pinch of ginger

Salt and pepper to taste

Directions

Salad

Rinse and pat dry spinach. Remove stems. Cut red peppers in half, remove seeds and membranes, and rinse clean. Slice into bite-size pieces. Blanch asparagus and cut into bite size pieces, discarding the bottom third of the stem. (To blanch, boil vegetable in water for 3 minutes, drain, and immerse in ice cold water. Drain again.) Slice cooked chicken into strips. Place all salad ingredients in a large bowl, excluding the cooked chicken and a few mandarin oranges. Toss with half of the chilled salad dressing.

Divide equally between four chilled plates. Top with sliced chicken and garnish with leftover mandarin oranges and optional feta or goat cheese. Serve balance of dressing on the side.

Dressing:

Whisk all ingredients together in a small bowl and chill until ready to serve (at least 30 minutes). Yields ³/₂ cup.

Nutritional Value Per Serving

Calories: 351
Total fat: 12 g
Saturated fat: 1.5 g
Protein: 24 g
Carbohydrate: 39 g
Sodium: 126 mg
% Fat: 29
% Protein: 30
% Carbohydrates: 41

10. Banana Berry Sundae

If you are a dessert lover, you'll want to try this healthful dairy-free alternative to a traditional sundae. Try a variety of fresh berries to liven up this dish. You'll wonder why you've waited so long to try a soy-based frozen dessert! We recommend, however, that you consume high-carbohydrate desserts in moderation, even if they contain healthful ingredients. Remember, the goal is to consume balanced, nutritious meals.

Serves: 4

Ingredients

$^3/_4$ cup fresh orange juice

1 teaspoon cinnamon

2 tablespoons pure maple sugar (optional)

4 cups vanilla flavored nondairy frozen dessert (look for a brand sweetened with brown rice syrup, not sugar)

1 banana

1 cup fresh berries

$^1/_4$ cup chopped walnuts

Directions

Whisk orange juice, cinnamon, and (optional) maple sugar in medium bowl. Spoon 1 cup of frozen soy into each bowl. Arrange berries over frozen soy and add sliced bananas. Drizzle orange juice mixture over the top and sprinkle with walnuts. Serve immediately.

Nutritional Value Per Serving

Calories: 238

Total fat: 8 g

Saturated fat: <1 g

Protein: 5 g

Carbohydrate: 39 g

Sodium: 55 mg

% Fat: 31

% Protein: 9

% Carbohydrates: 60

The Basics for Everyday Use

In addition to the top ten vitality recipes, the following recipes provide the basic "staples" for many healthful meals.

- Steamed Chicken Breasts (or Salmon)
- Everyday Chicken
- Chicken Stock
- Spiced Black Beans
- Perfectly Steamed Brown Rice
- Hummus (Mediterranean Spread)
- Tzatziki (Greek Cucumber Yogurt Sauce)

Steamed Chicken Breasts (or Salmon)
Serves: 4

Ingredients

4 boneless, organic skinless chicken breasts

2 tablespoons Cajun Creole Seasoning or other prepared seasoning of choice

Citrus salad dressing marinade (optional: see citrus spinach salad recipe)

Directions

Rinse chicken and remove excess skin and fat. Generously apply the seasoning or marinate in citrus salad dressing for 30 minutes in refrigerator or use immediately. When ready to cook, steam chicken in an electric steamer (such as a Krups Optisteam Plus Steamer) for 25 minutes. Serve whole, sliced, or shredded. (You can also prepare salmon this same way.)

Nutritional Value Per Serving:

Calories: 78

Total fat: <1 g

Saturated fat: <1 g

Protein: 16 g

Carbohydrate: 0 g

Sodium: 46 mg

% Fat: 10

% Protein: 90

% Carbohydrates: 0

Basic Sautéed Chicken

Serves: 4

Ingredients

4 boneless, organic skinless chicken breasts

3 teaspoons olive oil

Kosher salt

Fresh ground peppercorn blend

Granulated garlic

Directions

Wash and trim the chicken breast and pat dry. Drizzle with olive oil and rub onto both sides. Sprinkle lightly with kosher salt, pepper, and garlic. Let chicken sit for a few minutes for flavors to develop or if in a hurry use immediately.

Using a nonstick sauté pan or non-stick ridged grill pan, spray lightly with olive oil–flavored nonstick spray and bring to medium heat. Add chicken breasts to hot pan and cook until both sides are well caramelized and a toasty golden color. Depending on size and thickness of chicken breasts, this will take just a few minutes per side.

Remove from heat and enjoy it plain, in a salad, or add a healthful sauce of your choice.

Nutritional Value Per Serving

Calories: 195

Total fat: 6 g

Saturated fat: 1 g

Protein: 33 g

Carbohydrate: 0 g

Sodium: 92 mg

% Fat: 30

% Protein: 70

% Carbohydrates: 0

Chicken Stock

Yields: 2 Quarts

Ingredients

2 pounds organic chicken with bones, excess skin and fat removed

4 carrots, roughly chopped into 1-inch pieces

4 onions, roughly chopped into 1-inch pieces

4 celery stalks, roughly chopped into 1-inch pieces

3 cloves garlic, peeled

10 peppercorns

1 bay leaf

$^1/_2$ cup chopped parsley, stems included

cold filtered water

Directions

Place all ingredients in a stockpot large enough to hold
everything easily. Cover with cold filtered water. Bring
to a boil over high heat. Reduce the heat and skim off
any foam or fat that rises to the surface. Simmer for at
least 2 hours, uncovered. Strain and cool quickly.
Refrigerate. When the stock is thoroughly chilled, fat
will rise to the top and solidify. Remove the solid fat
and discard it. Salt and pepper to taste. Use within 4
days, or freeze leftover stock.

Nutritional Value Per Serving ($^1/_2$ cup)

Calories: 20

Total fat: <1 g

Saturated fat: <1 g

Protein: 4 g

Carbohydrate: 2 g

Sodium: 330 mg

% Fat: 5

% Protein: 70

% Carbohydrates: 25

Spiced Black Beans

For a faster preparation, beans can be heated through in the pan with the tomatoes and spices, but be careful to stir gently as not to break up the beans. This could be topped with a dollop of nonfat sour cream and a slice of avocado. These beans work well as a side dish or as a base for healthy soft tacos or a layered Mexican torte.

Serves: 4-6

Ingredients

1 tablespoon olive oil

3 cloves garlic, finely minced

$1/2$ cup chopped red onion

2 teaspoons ground cumin

1 15-ounce can diced tomatoes, drained and chopped lightly

2 15-ounce cans black beans, rinsed and drained

2 tablespoons chopped cilantro

Kosher salt and fresh pepper to taste

Directions

Preheat oven to 325 degrees.

In a small nonstick pan over medium heat, add oil, garlic, and onion and sauté for about 5 minutes until onion is soft and translucent, being careful not to burn garlic. Add cumin and sauté 1 to 2 minutes. Add tomato and stir until combined, sautéing a few more minutes.

Pour into a small baking dish and gently stir in beans. Cover and heat through in preheated oven, about 20 minutes. Stir in cilantro just before serving.

Nutritional Value Per Serving
  Calories: 132
  Total fat: 2.6 g
  Saturated fat: <1 g
  Protein: 6 g
  Carbohydrate: 24 g
  Sodium: 484 mg
  % Fat: 16
  % Protein: 19
  % Carbohydrates: 65

Perfectly Steamed Brown Rice
  Serves: 4–6

Ingredients:
  1 cup brown rice (short grain or basmati)
  1 cup homemade chicken or vegetable stock, or pre-
      pared organic low-sodium chicken or vegetable
      broth
  1 tablespoon spice mixture (recommend The Spice
      Hunter Seafood Grill and Broil if serving rice with
      fish or Cajun Creole Seasoning if serving with
      chicken or for use in soups or chicken rollups)
  Onion and button mushrooms, chopped (optional)

Directions
  Recommend using a Krups Optisteam Plus Steamer. If
  not using an electric steamer, follow directions on the

rice package. For steaming, fill water reservoir to maximum fill line. Rinse brown rice 2 to 3 times to remove dust and "bad" rice pieces. Combine all ingredients in rice bowl. If adding onions and mushrooms, sauté first and reduce liquid before adding to rice to compensate for the liquid mushrooms will release during steaming process. Put rice bowl in steaming tray and cover with the lid. Set timer to 55 minutes. Fluff rice with fork and serve.

Nutritional Value Per Serving:

Calories: 17
Total fat: 1.50 g
Saturated fat: 0 g
Protein: 3.25 g
Carbohydrate: 34 g
Sodium: 142 mg
% Fat: 8
% Protein: 8
% Carbohydrates: 84

Hummus (Mediterranean Spread)

Serves: 10

Ingredients

15-ounce can garbanzo beans (chickpeas)
1 tablespoon tahini (sesame paste)
2 tablespoon lemon juice
1 teaspoon finely chopped garlic
4 tablespoons olive oil
$\frac{1}{2}$ teaspoon red pepper (optional)
Salt and freshly ground pepper to taste

Directions

Drain and rinse garbanzo beans. Puree them in a blender or food processor with the tahini, lemon juice, red pepper, and garlic. With the machine running, pour the olive oil slowly through the opening in the lid until the hummus becomes thick and creamy. Add salt and pepper to taste. Serve with sprouted-grain or whole-wheat pita bread. (Store the remaining hummus in a covered container in the refrigerator for up to 5 days.)

Nutritional Value Per Serving

Calories: 141
Total fat: 5 g
Saturated fat: 1 g
Protein: 6 g
Carbohydrate: 18 g
Sodium: 104 mg
% Fat: 33
% Protein: 18
% Carbohydrates: 49

Tzatziki (Greek Cucumber Sauce)

Serves: 4–6

Ingredients

1 cup nonfat plain yogurt
1 cup nonfat (or low-fat) sour cream
1 large cucumber
$\frac{1}{2}$ cup lemon juice and zest of one-half of a lemon
$\frac{1}{2}$ teaspoon salt

2 tablespoons fresh dill

1 fresh garlic clove

Directions

Peel cucumber and slice in quarters, lengthwise. Remove seeds. Place cucumber slices in plastic bag and add sea salt (this will expel the excess water in the cucumber) for 30 minutes. Remove cucumber from bag and pat dry with paper towel. Chop into small pieces. Squeeze and eliminate any excess water from chopped cucumber pieces.

Combine yogurt, sour cream, lemon juice, lemon zest, dill, and minced garlic. Fold in cucumber. Allow to marinate for several hours before serving. Keeps well refrigerated for a week.

Nutritional Value Per Serving

Calories: 66

Total fat: 1 g

Saturated fat: <1 g

Protein: 4 g

Carbohydrate: 13 g

Sodium: 47 mg

% Fat: 1

% Protein: 23

% Carbohydrates: 76

Appendix F
Detoxification and Elimination Diet

We suggest you take the Medical Symptom Questionnaire (MSQ) that follows on page 308 from Metagenics, Inc., to identify your need for detoxification. Scores of 75 or more on the MSQ suggest that you will benefit from a detoxification program. Detoxification requires you to be on the elimination diet outlined below; this will eliminate the most common allergenic foods. Additionally, you will need to eliminate all foods that you crave, as you may actually be allergic to them; craving is one indication of a food allergy.

We recommend detoxification with either UltraClear PLUS® or UltraInflamX from Metagenics, Inc. If you have many digestive tract symptoms listed on the MSQ, or if you score six or higher, UltraInflamX is suggested. If you have frequent problems with joints and muscle aches and pains and stiffness, or have symptoms of eczema or hives, UltraInflamX is also suggested. Otherwise, UltraClear PLUS can be used for detoxification. Both these products have ample amounts of protein to support liver detoxification. UltraClear PLUS specifically has more nutrients to support the liver. UltraInflamX has specific ingredients to reduce inflammation.

If you score between 50 to 100 on the MSQ, use UltraClear PLUS or UltraInflamX three times daily for two weeks, then consume two scoops three times a day for one week.

If you score over 100 on the MSQ, use UltraClear PLUS or UltraInflamX, one-half scoop three times a day for one week, then one scoop three times a day for one week. Follow with UltraClear PLUS, two scoops three times daily for two weeks, or UltraInflamX, two scoops two times daily for two weeks.

Alkaline Broth

The following alkaline broth is very helpful to use during the detoxification process. It has very little allergenic potential and the nutrients aid in detoxification. During detoxification, you need to eat five or six small meals per day. A minimum of 1,000 to 1,200 caloric intake each day is important. Unless you are sensitive to them, multivitamin and minerals supplementation is suggested during detoxification program.

Directions

Place equal amounts of the following vegetables in a steamer basket: spinach, zucchini, parsley, celery, and green beans. Make sure that the steamer basket remains above the level of the water at all times. Steam the vegetables, testing them with a fork to ensure that they do not become soft. Remove the vegetables from the steamer while still crunchy. Place the vegetables and the water in which you steamed them into a blender. Puree the mixture in the blender, adding your favorite herbs (such as basil, garlic, or dill) for flavor. Drink eight ounces of this alkaline broth for the first few days during detoxification.

MEDICAL SYMPTOMS QUESTIONNAIRE

Rate each of the following symptoms based on your typical health profile for the past thirty days.

Scoring Key

0 = never or almost never have the symptom

1 = occasionally have it, effect is not severe

2 = occasionally have it, effect is severe

3 = frequently have it, effect is not severe

4 = frequently have it, effect is severe

Area	Symptom	Point (0, 1, 2, 3, 4)
Head	Headaches	
	Faintness	
	Dizziness	
	Insomnia	
		Total:
Eyes	Watery or itchy eyes	
	Swollen, reddened, sticky eyelids	
	Bags or dark circles under eyes	
	Blurred or tunnel vision (does not include near or far-sightedness	
		Total:
Ears	Itchy ears	
	Earaches, eat infections	
	Drainage from ear	
	Ringing in ears, hearing loss	
		Total:
Nose	Stuffy nose	
	Sinus problems	
	Hay fever	
	Sneezing attacks	
	Excessive mucus formation	
		Total:

Mouth/Throat	Chronic coughing	
	Gagging, frequent need to clear throat	
	Sore throat, hoarseness, loss of voice	
	Swollen or discolored tongue, gums, lips	
	Canker sores	
		Total:
Skin	Acne	
	Hives, rashes, dry skin	
	Hair loss	
	Flushing, hot flashes	
	Excessive sweating	
		Total:
Heart	Irregular or skipped heartbeat	
	Rapid or pounding heartbeat	
	Chest pain	
		Total:
Lungs	Cheat congestion	
	Asthma, bronchitis	
	Shortness of breath	
	Difficulty breathing	
		Total:
Digestive Tract	Nausea, vomiting	
	Diarrhea	
	Constipation	
	Bloating feeling Belching, passing gas	
	Heartburn	
	Intestinal/stomach pain	
		Total:

Joints/Muscle	Pain or aches in joints	
	Arthritis	
	Stiffness or limitation of movement	
	Pain or aches in muscles	
	Feeling of weakness or tiredness	
		Total:
Weight	Binge eating/drinking	
	Craving certain foods	
	Excessive weight	
	Compulsive eating	
	Water retention	
	Underweight	
		Total:
Energy/Activity	Fatigue, sluggishness	
	Apathy, lethargy	
	Hyperactivity	
	Restlessness	
		Total:
Mind	Poor memory	
	Confusion, poor comprehension	
	Poor concentration	
	Poor physical coordination	
	Difficulty in making decisions	
	Stuttering or stammering	
	Slurred speech	
	Learning disabilities	
		Total:
Emotions	Mood swings	
	Anxiety, fear, nervousness	
	Anger, irritability, aggressiveness	
	Depression	
		Total:

Other	Frequent illness	
	Frequent or urgent urinations	
	Genital itch or discharge	
		Total:
		Grand Total:

Refer to the introduction of this Appendix for recommendations.

Modified Elimination Diet—To Be Used During Detoxification

This dietary approach has been most helpful in patients who complain of recurrent gastrointestinal problems, especially diarrhea, food intolerance or sensitivity, chemical or environmental sensitivities, and chronic headache of unknown etiology.

You may feel worse for four to five days, and then feel better. The diet needs to be continued for at least three to four weeks for improvements to be stabilized. After symptoms have subsided, you need to work with a health practitioner to add some foods back slowly. Some people with many food allergies need to do food allergy testing (see Appendix B). The Modified Elimination diet is low-lactose, low-fat, gluten-free, and usually well tolerated. A summary of the dietary guidelines is outlined below.

The primary guidelines are:

1. Eliminate dairy products such as milk, cheese, and ice cream. *(Note: Varying amounts of natural, unsweetened, live-culture yogurt may be tolerated by some individuals.)*
2. Avoid meats such as beef, pork, or veal. Chicken, turkey, lamb, and cold-water fish, such as salmon, mackerel, and

halibut, are acceptable if you are not allergic to these foods. Select free-range poultry whenever possible.

3. Eliminate gluten. Avoid any food that contains wheat, spelt, kamut, oats, rye, barley, amaranth, quinoa or malts. This is the most difficult part of the diet but also the most important. Unfortunately, gluten is contained in many common foods such as bread, crackers, pasta, cereals, and products containing flour made from these grains. Corn is also a common allergen and should be avoided. Products made from rice, buckwheat, gluten-free flour, potato, tapioca, and arrowroot may be used as desired by most individuals.

4. Drink at least two quarts of water, preferable filtered, daily.

5. Avoid all alcohol-containing products including beer, wine, liquor, and over-the-counter products that contain alcohol. Also avoid all caffeine-containing beverages including coffee, caffeinated tea, and soft drinks. Coffee substitutes from gluten-containing grains should also be avoided along with decaffeinated coffee.

Read labels carefully, as over-the-counter medications may contain alcohol and/or caffeine.

ELIMINATION DIET SUMMARY

Food Group	Allowed	Avoid
Protein	Chicken, turkey, lamb All legumes, dried peas, and lentils Cold-water fish such as salmon, halibut, and mackerel	Red meats, cold cuts, frankfurters, sausage, canned sausage, canned meats, eggs
Dairy Products	Unsweetened, live-culture yogurt Milk substitutes such as rice milk, nut milks, and soy beverages	Milk, cheese, ice-cream, cream, nondairy creamers
Starch	White or sweet potato, rice tapioca, buckwheat, and gluten-free products,	All products containing gluten (including pasta)
Soups	Clear vegetable-based broth, homemade vegetarian soups	Canned or cream soups
Vegetables	All vegetables, preferably fresh, frozen, or freshly juiced	Creamed or in casseroles
Beverages	Unsweetened fruit or vegetable, juices, water, non citrus herbal tea	Milk, coffee, tea, cocoa, Postum, alcoholic beverages, sodas, sweetened beverages, citrus juices
Bread/Cereals	Any made from rice, corn, buckwheat, millet, soy, potato flour, tapioca, arrow root, or gluten-free flour products	All made from wheat, oat, spelt, kamut, rye, barley, amaranth, quinoa, or gluten
Fruits	Unsweetened fresh, frozen, or water-packed, canned fruits excluding citrus and strawberries	Fruit drinks, lemonade, citrus, strawberries, dried fruit
Fats/Oils/Nuts	Cold/expeller-pressed, unrefined, flaxseed oil, olive oil, and sunflower oil, ghee, sunflower seeds, sesame dressings/seeds, flax seeds,pumpkin seeds, squash seeds/butters, salad dressings made from allowed ingredients, almonds, cashews, pecans, walnuts	Margarine, shortening, unclarified butter, refined oils, peanuts, salad spreads made from ingredients in the avoid column

Appendix G
Understanding Nutrition Facts Labels

Although the example highlighted below is for cookies, we are not recommending that you eat cookies; if you choose to indulge in moderation, we suggest you consume nutritious cookies made with rolled oats, whole-wheat flower, and a healthier sugar substitute such as fructose or xylitol.

It is important to note that prepackaged or convenience foods may present the nutritional information as "as-packaged" values; any additional ingredients you need to prepare the food are not included.

Serving Size

The nutritional information provided is based on the serving size listed. For example, the serving size shown here is three cookies (33g). If you consume six cookies, the nutritional values provided need to be doubled.

Cookies
Nutrition Facts

Serving Size 3 Cookies (33g)
Servings per container About 17

Amount per serving
Calories 160
　Calories from fat 60

	% Daily Value
Total Fat 7.0g	10%
Saturated Fat 1.5 g	7%
Polyunsaturated Fat 0.5g	
Monosaturated Fat 3g	
Cholesteral 0mg	0%
Sodium 220mg	9%
Total Carbohydrate 23g	7%
Dietary Fiber 1g	4%
Sugars 13g	
Protein 1g	
Vitamin A	0%
Vitamin C	0%
Calcium	0%
Iron	8%

* Percentage Daily Values are based on a 2,000 calorie diet. Your daily values may be higher or lower depending on your caloric needs.:

		Calories 2,000	2,600
Total Fat	Less than	66g	80g
Sat. Fat	Less than	20g	25g
Cholesterol	Less than	300mg	300mg
Sodium	Less than	2,400mg	2,400mg
Total Carbohydrate		300g	375g
Dietary Fiber		25g	30g

Calories per gram:
Fat 9   Carbohydrate 4   Protein 4

Ingredients: SUGAR, ENRICHED WHEAT FLOUR (CONTAINS NIACIN, REDUCED IRON THIAMINE, MONONITRATE, RIBOFLAVIN, FOLIC ACID), VEGETABLE SHORTENING, PARTIALLY HYDROGENATED SOYBEAN OIL, COCOA, HIGH FRUCTOSE CORN SYRUP, CORN FLOUR, WHEY, CORNSTARCH, BAKING SODA, SOY LECITHIN, VANILLA, CHOCOLATE.

Calories, Calories from Fat

This information helps you monitor the number of calories you take in each day. More important, it allows you to make healthy decisions about the foods you eat. In this example, 39 percent of the calories come from fat—anything over 30 percent is probably too much.

If the calories from fat are not listed on an ingredient label, you can estimate the percentage of fat calories by multiplying the total fat grams by 9 and divide the sum by the total calories. You can apply this formula to determine the percentage of calories for protein and carbohydrates; however, you will use 4, instead of 9, as your multiplier.

In this example, the calories from fat are 60. Divide this number by the total calories (160) to calculate the approximate percentage of fat, which is 37 percent.

Total Fat, Saturated Fat

Choose products that are devoid of saturated fats and trans fats, both of which are linked to an early onset of cardiovascular disease and increase other health risks. Keep your consumption of saturated fat to less than 5 percent of your daily caloric intake.

Although trans fat isn't listed on the label, foods containing hydrogenated or partially hydrogenated ingredients contain trans fat, which is known to increase LDL (bad) cholesterol levels. In contrast, foods containing monounsaturated fats, such as olive oil, are actually good for you. To calculate trans fat, add the saturated, polyunsaturated, and monounsaturated fats together and subtract from the total fat. This is likely the amount of hidden trans fat in the food. In this example, the amount of trans fat is 2.0 grams.

Cholesterol

Use this information to reduce the aging of your arteries. Limit your dietary cholesterol intake to less than 125 milligrams per 1,000 calories.

Sodium

The American Heart Association recommends a diet that contains no more than 2,400 milligrams of sodium each day. To reduce the amount of sodium in your diet, avoid high-sodium foods such as processed meats, canned soups, and snack foods such as potato chips.

Total Carbohydrate

When you choose carbohydrates, make them complex or low glycemic. Look for words such as "whole grain" or "100 percent whole wheat" as the first ingredient on the product label. The words "healthy" or "multigrain" do not ensure a whole-grain food. We suggest 40 to 50 percent of your daily calories come from carbohydrates.

Dietary Fiber

Use this information on the food label to keep track of how much fiber is in your diet—we suggest at least 40 grams per day.

Sugars

All sugars are not created equal. Refined and simple sugars create a number of health risks. Limit these sugars to less than 5 percent of your total daily caloric intake.

Protein

You can get protein from animal products, such as eggs, meat, or cheese, or from vegetable sources, such as soy products, nuts, legumes and beans, and seeds.

A diet high in vegetable proteins is much more beneficial. By themselves, the vegetable protein sources listed above contain fewer amino acids (the building blocks of proteins) than meats, but when you combine these sources with whole grains, such as brown rice, barley, and wheat, all your protein needs can be met.

We suggest 20 to 30 percent of your daily calories come from protein.

Vitamins and Minerals

This section of the label gives you the information you need to determine the amount of valuable nutrients available in the product. As you can see from this label, cookies offer virtually no nutritional value.

Percent Daily Values

Based on a 2,000-calorie per day diet, the percent daily value (%DV) calculates the nutrition facts using a percentage. This makes it easy to determine how much of the recommended daily intake of a nutrient is in each serving of food. Please refer to Appendix C, which lists our nutritional recommendations for optimum health.

Ingredients

Ingredients are listed in order by the relative concentration of that ingredient. Look at the first, second, third, and fourth items in the list of ingredients. If any of the first four lists a saturated fat, a partially hydrogenated vegetable oil, a simple sugar, a non-whole-grain carbohydrate, or salt, we recommend you avoid this product.

Appendix H
References

Chapter 1

1. *National Vital Statistics Reports*, 49(12): 40 pps., (PHS) 2001–1120.

2. P. H. Bennett, "Type 2 Diabetes among the Pima Indians of Arizona: An Epidemic Attributable to Environmental Change?," *Nutrition Reviews*, 1999; 57(5): S51–S54.

3. J. V. Neel, The 'Thrifty Genotype," *Nutrition Reviews*, 1999; 57(5): S2–S9.

4. P. :ichtenstein et al.,*New England Journal of Medicine*, 2000; 343(2):78-85.

5. Great Smokies Diagnostic Laboratory Comprehensive Cardiovascular Profile 2.0.

6. C. G. Su et al., "A Novel Therapy for Colitis Utilizing PPARg Ligands to Inhibit the Epithelial Inflammatory Response," *Journal of Clinical Investigation*, 1999; 104(4): 383–89.

7. H. R. Superko and H. S. Hecht, "Metabolic disorders contribute to subclinical coronary atherosclerosis in patients with coronary calcification." *American Journal of Cardiology*, 2001; 88: 260–64.

8. P. Bavenhalm et al., *Metabolism*, 1995; 44(11): 1481–88.

9. H. N. Hodis et al., "Intermediate-density lipoproteins and progression of carotid arterial wall intima-media thickness." *Circulation*, 1997; 95(8): 2022–6.

10. W. J. Mack, R. M. Krauss, and H. N. Hodis, "Lipoprotein subclasses in the Monitored Atherosclerosis Regression Study (MARS). Treatment effects and relation to coronary angiographic progression." *Arteriosclerosis, Thrombosis, and Vascular Biology*, 1996; 16(5): 697–704.

11. G. R. Thompson, "Angiographic evidence for the role of triglyceride-rich lipoproteins in progression of coronary artery disease." *European Heart Journal*, 1998; 19 Suppl H: H31–6.

12. H. R. Superko, "Did grandma give you heart disease? The new battle against coronary artery disease." *American Journal of Cardiology*, 1998; 82: 34Q–46Q.

13. A. C. St. Pierre et al.,"Comparison of various electrophoretic characteristics of LDL particles and their relationship to the risk of ischemic heart disease." *Circulation*, 2001; 104: 2295–9.

14. R. Ross, *In the Heart, Arteries, and Veins* (New York: McGraw-Hill, 1990), 106–11.

15. A. L. Miller and G. S. Kelly, *Alternative Medicine Review*, 1997; 2(4): 234–54.

16. E. A. Ashley, J. Myers, and V. Froelicher, "Exercise Testing in Clinical Medicine," *Lancet*, 2000; 356: 1592–97.

17. E. O. Nishime et al., "Heart Rate Recovery and Treadmill Exercise Score as Predictors of Mortality in Patients Referred for Exercise ECG," *Journal of the American Medical Association*, 2000; 284: 1392–98.

18. D. B. Mark et al., "Exercise Treadmill Score for Predicting Prognosis in Coronary Artery Disease," *Annals of Internal Medicine*, 1987; 106: 793–800.

19. C. R. Cole et al., "Heart Rate Recovery Immediately after Exercise as a Predictor of Mortality," *New England Journal of Medicine*, 1999; 341: 1351–57.

20. S. N. Blair, H. W. Kohl III, and R. S. Paffenbarger et al., "Physical Fitness and All-Cause Mortality: A Prospective Study of Healthy Men and Women," *Journal of the American Medical Association*, 1989; 262: 2395–401.

21. S. N. Blair et al., "Influences of Cardio Respiratory Fitness and Other Precursors on Cardiovascular Disease and All-Cause Mortality in Men and Women," *Journal of the American Medical Association*, 1996; 276: 205–10.

22. B. Ames, Proceedings of the National Academy of Sciences: University of California at Berkeley, 1993.

23. L. G. Russek and G. E. Schwartz, "Perceptions of Parental Caring Predict Health Status in Midlife: A 35-Year Follow-up of the Harvard Mastery of Stress Study," *Psychosomatic Medicine*, 1997; 59(2): 144-149.

24. D. Funkenstein, S. King, and M. Drollet, *Mastery of Stress* (Cambridge, MA: Harvard University Press, 1957).

Chapter 2

1. A. I. Terr, et al., "Environmental illness. A clinical review of 50 cases." *Archives of Internal Medicine*, 1986; 146: 145–9.

2. D. A. Mrazek and M. Klinnert, "Asthma: Psychoneuroimmunologic Considerations," in R. Ader, ed., *Psychoneuroimmunlogy* 2d ed. (Orlando, FL: Academic Press, 1990), 1013–35.

3. T. M. Dembroski et al., "Components of Hostility as Predictors of Sudden Death and Myocardial Infarction in the Multiple Risk Factor Intervention Trial," *Psychosomatic Medicine*, 1989; 51: 514–22.

4. R. B. Shekelle et al., "Hostility, Risk of Coronary Artery Disease and Mortality," *Psychosomatic Medicine*, 1983; 45: 109–114.

5. J. C. Barefoot, W. G. Dahlstrom, and R. B. Williams, "Hostility, CHD Incidence, and Total Mortality: A 25-Year Follow-Up Study of 255 Physicians," *Psychosomatic Medicine*, 1983; 45: 59–63.

6. C. Raymond, "Distrust, Rage May Be Toxic Core That Puts Type A Person at Risk," *Journal of the American Medical Association*, 1989; 261(16): 813.

7. K. Orth-Gomer and A. Unden, "Type A Behavior, Social Support, and Coronary Risk: Interaction and Significance for Mortality in Cardiac Patients," *Psychosomatic Medicine*, 1990; 52: 59–72.

8. S. G. Haynes and M. Frankenhaeser, "Type A Behavior, Employment Status, and Coronary Heart Disease in Women," *Behavioral Medicine Update*, 1984; 6(4): 11–15.

9. H. Weiner, "Rheumatoid Arthritis," *Psychobiology and Human Disease*, 1977; 416–94; J. S. Heisel, "Life Changes as Etiologic Factors in Juvenile Rheumatoid Arthritis," *Journal of Psychosomatic Research*, 1972; 17: 411–20.

10. K. O. Anderson et al., "Rheumatoid Arthritis: Review of Psychological Factors Related to Etiology, Effects, and Treatment," *Psychological Bulletin*, 1985; 98: 358–87.

11. L. F. Callahan et al., "Further Analysis of Learned Helplessness in Rheumatoid Arthritis using a Rheumatology Attitudes Index," *Journal of Rheumatology*, 1988; 15: 418–26.

12. H. Dreher, "The Type C Connection: A Powerful New Tool in the Fight Against Cancer," in Proceedings of the Fourth National Conference on the Psychology of Health, Immunity, and Disease, National Institute for the Clinical Application of Behavioral Medicine.

13. B. Brower, "The Character of Cancer," *Science News*, 1987; 131: 120–21.

14. R. S. Surwit et al., "Stress and Diabetes Mellitus," *Diabetes Care*, 1992; 15: 1413–22.

15. "Mind/Hypertension Link Certain, Researchers Say," *Brain/Mind Bulletin*, July 1989, 2.

16. M. Camilleri and C. M. Prather, "The Irritable Bowel Syndrome," *Annals of Internal Medicine*, 1992; 116: 1001–1008.

17. S. Cohen and G. M. Williamson, "Stress and Infectious Disease in Humans," *Psychological Bulletin*, 1991; 109: 5–24.

18. M. Antoni, *Mind Body Medicine* (Needham Heights, MA: Allyn & Bacon, 1996), 24.

19. S.C. Kobasa, "How Much Stress Can You Survive?," *American Health*, September 1984, 67.

20. D. Shapiro, *Control Therapy* (New York: John Wiley and Sons, 1998).

21. U. L. Gonik et al., "Cost Effectiveness of Behavioral Medicine Procedures in the Treatment of Stress-Related Disorders," *Journal of Clinical Biofeedback*, 1981; 4: 16–24.

22. D. W. Orme-Johnson, L. Domash, and E. Farrow, *Scientific Research on Transcendental Meditation, Collected Papers*, vol. 1 (Los Angeles: MIU Press, 1974).

23. L. Sagan, *The Health of Nations* (New York: Basic Books, 1987), 137; M. Argyle, *The Psychology of Happiness* (London: Methuen and Co., 1987), 196.

Chapter 3

1. "Marriage and Wellness Linked," *Deseret News*, November 15, 1988, 4A.

2. R. T. Segraves, "Divorce and Health Problems," *Medical Aspects of Human Sexuality*, June 1989, 106.

3. B. R. Sarason, I. G. Sarason, and G. R. Pierce, *Social Support: An Interactional View* (New York: John Wiley and Sons, 1990), 257.

4. M. Pilisuk and S. Hiller Parks, *The Healing Web* (Hanover, NH: The University Press of New England, 1986).

5. J. A. Tooley and L. Y. Anderson, "Living Is Risky," *U.S. News and World Report*, January 25, 1988, 77.

6. A. Rosengren, H. Wedel, and L. Wilemson, "Marital Status and Mortality in the Middle Aged Swedish Men," *American Journal of Epidemiology*, 1989; 129(1): 54–64.

7. C. Turkington, "Have You Hugged Your Immune System Today?," *Self,* October 1988, 184.

8. M. Hunt, "Long-Life Insurance: For Men, It's Marriage," *Longevity,* February 1991, 10.

9. J. J. Lynch, *The Broken Heart: The Medical Consequences of Loneliness* (New York: Basic Books, 1977).

10. Ibid.

11. Hunt, "Long-Life Insurance," 10.

12. Sarason, Sarason, and Pierce, *Social Support,* 257.

13. Turkington, "Have You Hugged Your Immune System Today?," 184.

14. B. Powell, *Alone, Alive, and Well* (Emmaus, PA: Rodale Press, 1985).

15. Sarason, Sarason, and Pierce, *Social Support,* 257.

16. Powell, *Alone, Alive, and Well.*

17. S. Faelten, D. Diamond, and the editors of *Prevention Magazine, Take Control of Your Life: A Complete Guide to Stress Relief,* (Emmaus, PA: *Rodale Press,* 1988), 143–44.

18. R. Weiss, "Worried Sick: Hassles and Herpes," *Science News,* 1987; 132: 360.

19. J. K. Kiecolt-Glaser et al., "Marital Quality, Marital Disruption, and Immune Function," *Psychosomatic Medicine,* 1987; 49: 13–34.

20. Sarason, Sarason, and Pierce, *Social Support,* 257.

21. Powell, *Alone, Alive, and Well.*

22. M. Argyle, *The Psychology of Happiness* (New York: Methuen and Co., 1987).

23. "Communication with Spouse Reduces Cardiac Risk," *Brain/Mind and Common Sense,* 1992; 17(12): 1.

24. N. S. Jacobsen, A. Holtzworth-Monroe, and K. B. Schmaling, "Marital Therapy and Spouse Involvement in the Treatment of Depression, Agoraphobia, and Alcoholism," *Journal of Consulting/Clinical Psychology,* 1989; 1: 5–10.

25. C. Houck, "Under Covering the Secrets of Happiness," *Cosmopolitan,* n.d., 236–40.

26. B. Burman and G. Margolin, "Marriage and Health," *Advances,* 6(4): 1989, 51–58.

27. *Psychosomatic Medicine,* 1993; 55: 395-409.

28. L. Murray, "Mad Marriages: Arguing Your Way to Better Health," *Longevity,* October 1993, 29. Faelten et al.*, Take Control of Your Life,* 143–44.

30. J. H. Medalie and U. Goldburt, "Angina Pectoris among 10,000 Men: Psychosocial and Other Risk Factors as Evidenced by a Multivariate Analysis of a Five Year Incidence Study," *American Journal of Medicine*, 1976; 60(6): 910–21.

31. Lynch, *The Broken Heart*.

32. G. E. Rodgers, "Communication with Spouse," *Brain/Mind and Common Sense*, 1.

33. J. Gottman, *The Marriage Clinic* (New York: W.W. Norton & Co., 1999), 45.

34. S. Witelson, "Hand and Sex Differences in the Isthmus and Anterior Commissure of the Human Corpus Callosum," *Brain*, 1989; 112: 799–835; A. Moin and D. Jessel, *Brain Sex* (New York: Dell, 1989).

35. D. Blum, *Sex on the Brain: The Biological Differences Between Men and Women* (New York: Viking, 1997).

36. J. Jampolsky, *Love is Letting Go of Fear* (Berkeley, CA: Celestial Arts Publishing, 1979), 69.

Chapter 6

1. JAMA, June 19, 2002: Two studies support the use of dietary supplements in healthy adults to reduce the risk of cancer, heart disease, and osteoporosis. This is the first time the American Medical Association endorsed the use of dietary supplements in preventing disease.

2. In April 2001, the famous Nurses' Health Study in the *Harvard Women's Health Watch Journal* reported that women who took folic acid in multivitamins for at least fifteen years were 75 percent less likely to develop colon cancer.

3. U.S. Government of Health Services: Centers for Disease Control and Prevention, "Dietary Intakes of Vitamins, Minerals, and Fiber of Persons Ages 2 Months and over in the United States: Third National Health and Nutrition Examination Survey, Phase 1, 1988–91," *Public Health Service Publication*, 1994; 258.

4. M. M. Zive et al., "Marginal Vitamin and Mineral Intakes of Young Adults: The Bogalusa Heart Study," *Journal of Adolescent Health*, 1996; 19(1): 39–47.

5. G. Block and B. Abrams, "Vitamin and Mineral Status of Women of Childbearing Potential," *Annals of the New York Academy of Sciences*, 1993; 678: 244–54.

6. M. B. Reddy and M. Love, "The impact of food processing on the nutritional quality of vitamins and minerals" in Jackson, et al., ed., *Impact of Processing of Food Safety* (New York: Plenum Publishers, 1999).

7. D. V. Parke and C. Loannides, "The Role of Nutrition in Toxicology," *Annual Review of Nutrition,* 1981; 1: 207–34.

8. M. Brin, "Erythrocyte as a Biopsy Tissue for Functional Evaluation of Thiamine Adequacy," *Journal of the American Medical Association,* 1964; 187: 186–90.

9. B. N. Ames, "Micronutrient Deficiencies. A Major Cause of DNA Damage," *Annals of the New York Academy of Sciences,* 1999; 889: 87–106.

10. B. N. Ames and M. K. Shigenaga, "Oxidants Are a Major Contributor to Aging," *Annals of the New York Academy of Sciences,* 1992; 663: 85–96.

11. M. J. Richard and A. M. Roussel, "Micronutrients and Aging: Intakes and Requirements," *Proceedings of the Nutrition Society,* 1999; 58(3): 573–78.

12. J. Bland, "Guest Editorial: Beta-carotene Controversy," *Journal of Advancement in Medicine,* 1996; 9(2): 91–94.

13. H. D. Ashmead, "Comparative Intestinal Absorption and Subsequent Metabolism of Metal Amino Acid Chelates and Inorganic Metal Salts" in *Biological Trace Element Research: Multidisciplinary Perspectives,* ACS Symposium Series 445 (Washington, D.C.: American Chemical Society, 1991).

14. H. D. Ashmead, D. J. Graff, and H. H. Ashmead, *Intestinal Absorption of Metal Ions and Chelates* (Springfield, IL: Charles C. Thomas, 1985).

15. E. B. Rimm et al., "Folate and Vitamin B_6 from Diet and Supplements in Relation to Risk of Coronary Heart Disease among Women," *Journal of the American Medical Association,* 1998; 279: 359–64.

16. S. W. Hoag, H. Ramachandruni, and R. F. Shangraw, "Failure of Prescription Prenatal Vitamin Products to Meet USP Standards for Folic acid Dissolution," *Journal of the American Pharmaceutical Association,* 1997; NS37(4): 397–400.

17. M. K. Stamatakis and P. J. Meyer-Stout, "Disintegration Performance of Renal Multivitamin Supplements," *Journal of Renal Nutrition,* 1999; 9(2): 78–83.

Chapter 7

1. W. J. Vogelsang et al., "Intestinal Permeability and the Prediction of Relapse in Crohn's Disease," *Lancet*, 1993; 341: 1437–39

2. O. Martinez-Gonzalez et al., "Intestinal Permeability in Patients with Ankylosing Spondylitis and Their Healthy Relatives," *British Journal of Rheumatology*, 1994; 33: 644–47.

3. I. Bjarnason et al., "Intestinal Permeability in Patients with Celiac Disease and Dermatitis Herpetiforms," *Gut*, 1985; 26: 1214–19.

4. L. D. Juby et al. "Intestinal Permeability and Inflammation in Rheumatoid Arthritis," *British Journal of Rheumatology*, 1986; 25(2): 226–27.

5. E. S. Swenson, W. B. Milisen, and W. Curatolo, "Intestinal Permeability Enhancement: Efficacy, Acute Local Toxicity, and Reversibility," *Pharmaceutical Research*, 1994; 11(8): 1132–42.

6. J. Bland, "Applying New Essentials in Nutritional Medicine," *Healthcomm*, 1996: 162.

7. N. Kulkarni and B. S. Reddy, "Inhibitory Effect of Bifidobacterium Longum Cultures on the Azoxymethane-Induced Aberrant Crypt Foci Formation and Fecal Bacterial Betaglucuronidase," *Experimental Biology and Medicine*, 1994; 207: 278–83.

8. T. Mitsuoka, "Intestinal Flora and Aging," *Nutrition Reviews*, 1992; 50(12): 438–46.

9. J. O. Hunter, "Food Allergy—or Enterometabolic Disorder?," *Lancet*, 1991; 338: 495–96.

10. J. Egger et al., "Is Migraine Food Allergy?" *Lancet*, 1983; ii: 865–69.

11. V. Alun Jones et al. "Food Intolerance: A Major Factor in the Pathogenesis or Irritable Bowel Syndrome," *Lancet*, 1982; ii: 115–17.

12. V. Alun Jones et al., "Crohn's Disease: Maintenance of Remission by Diet," *Lancet*, 1985; ii: 177–80.

Chapter 9

1. J. D. Beasley and J. J. Swift, *The Kellogg Report*, Institute of Health Policy and Practice: Bard College Center, 1989; 4: 171.

2. U.S. Environmental Protection Agency, "Toxics in the Community: National and Local Perspectives," 1989 Toxics Release Inventory National Report, Office of Toxic Substances, Washington, D.C., 1991.

3. J. Timbrel, *Principles of Biochemical Toxicology* 2d ed. (Washington, D.C.: Taylor and Francis, 1992).

4. B. Helleman, "Multiple Chemical Sensitivity," *Chemical and Engineering News*, July 22, 1991; 26–42.

5. P. Rooney et al., "A Short Review of the Relationship Between Intestinal Permeability and Inflammatory Joint Disease," *Clinical and Experimental Rheumatology*, 1990; 8: 75–83.

6. M. D. Smith et al., "Abnormal Bowel Permeability in Ankylosing Spondylitis and Rheumatoid Arthritis," *Journal of Rheumatology*, 1985; 12: 299–305.

7. G. B. Steventon et al., "Xenobiotic Metabolism in Alzheimer's Disease," *Neurology*, 1990; 40: 1095–98.

8. J. Bland and J. A. Bralley, "Nutritional Up Regulation of Hepatic Detoxification Enzymes," *Journal of Applied Nutrition*, 1992; 44.

9. E. M. Boyd and C. P. Chen, "Lindane Toxicity and Protein-Deficient Diet," *Archives of Environmental Health*, 1968; 17: 156–63.

10. J. W. T. Dickerson et al., "Activity of Drug-Metabolizing Enzymes in the Liver of Growing Rats Fed on Diets High in Sucrose, Glucose, Fructose," *Proceedings of the Nutrition Society*, 1971; 30: 27A–28A.

11. M. J. Brodie et al., "Drug Metabolism in White Vegetarians," *British Journal of Clinical Pharmacology*, 1980; 9: 523–25.

12. K. E. Anderson and A. Kappas, "Dietary Regulation of Cytochrome P450," *Annual Review of Nutrition*, 1991; 11: 141–67.

Appendix I
Bibliography

Allardice, P. *The Art of Aromatherapy*. Avenel, NJ: Cresent Books/Random House, 1994.

Bland, J. *The 20-Day Rejuvenation Diet Program*. New Canaan, CT: Keats Publishing, 1996.

Brooks, G. A., and T. D. Fahey. *Exercise Physiology: Human Bioenergetics and Its Applications*. New York: Macmillan, 1984.

Brooks, G. A., and T. D. Fahey. *Fundamentals of Human Performance*. New York: Macmillan, 1987.

Carper, J. *Food: Your Miracle Medicine*. New York: HarperCollins, 1993.

Casdorph. J., and M. Walker. *Toxic Metal Syndrome: How Metal Poisonings Can Affect Your Brain*. Garden City Park, NY: Avery Publishing Group, 1995.

Chopra, D. *Ageless Body, Timeless Mind*. New York: Three Rivers Press, 1993.

Colgan, M. *Hormonal Health*. Vancouver, Canada: Apple Publishing, 1996

D'Adamo, P. J., and C. Whitney. *Eat Right for Your Type*. New York: G. P. Putnam's Sons, 1996.

Daoust, J., and G. Daoust. *40-30-30 Fat Burning Nutrition*. Del Mar, CA: Wharton Publishing, 1996.

DeLorme, R., and F. Stransky. *Fitness and Fallacies*. Dubuque, IA: Kendall/Hunt Publishing Co., 1990.

Ditchek, S. H. et al. *Healthy Child, Whole Child*. New York: HarperCollins, 2001.

Edell, D. E*at, Drink and Be Merry*. New York: HarperCollins, 1999.

Fahey, T. D. *Basic Weight Training*. Mountain View, CA: Mayfield Publishing Co., 1989.

Fahey, T. D., and G. Hutchinson. *Weight Training for Women*. Mountain View, CA: Mayfield Publishing Co., 1992.

Galland, L. P*ower Healing*. New York: Random House, 1998

Goldbeck, N., and D. Goldbeck. *The Healthiest Diet in the World: A Cookbook and Mentor*. New York: Dutton, 1998.

Gray, J. *Men Are from Mars, Women Are from Venus*. New York: HarperCollins, 1992.

Gray, J. M*en, Women and Relationships*. Hillsboro, OR: Beyond Words Publishing, 1993.

Haas, E. M. *The Detox Diet*. Berkeley, CA: Celestial Arts Publishing, 1996.

Hayes, D. *7 Habits of Healthy Aging*. San Clemente, CA: Innovative Practice Solutions, 2001.

Henner, M., and L. Henner. *Healthy Kids*. New York: HarperCollins, 2001.

Holford, P. *The Optimum Nutrition Bible*. Freedom, CA: The Crossing Press, 1999.

Holmes, T.H. and Rahe, R.H. The Social Readjustment Rating Scale. *Journal of Psychosomatic Research*, 1967. 11, 213-218.

Jensen, B. *Guide to Body Chemistry and Nutrition*. Los Angeles: Keats Publishing, 2000.

Jensen, B. *Nature Has a Remedy*. Los Angeles: Keats Publishing, 2001.

Jensen, B. *Nutrition Handbook: A Daily Regimen for Healthy Living*. Lincolnwood, IL: Keats Publishing, 2000.

McCully, K. *The Homocysteine Revolution*. New Caanan, CN: Keats Publishing, 1997.

Murray, M., and J. Pizzorno. *Encyclopedia of Natural Medicine*. Roseville, CA: Prima Publishing, 1998.

Northrup, C. *The Wisdom of Menopause*. New York: Bantam Books, 2001.

Padus, E. *The Complete Guide to Your Emotions and Your Health*. Emmaus, PA: Rodale Press, Inc., 1992.

Percival, M. *Functional Dietetics*. Colorado Springs, CO: Health Coach, 1995

Percival, M. *Take Charge of Your Health*. Colorado Springs, CO: Health Coach, 1996.

Percival, M. *Teaming Up for a Healthier You*. New Hamburg, Ontario: Health Coach Systems, 1995.

Perricone, N. *The Wrinkle Cure*. New York: Warner Books, 2001.

Phillips, B., and M. D'Orso. *Body for Life*. New York: HarperCollins, 1999.

Pirello, C. *Cooking the Whole Foods Way*. New York: The Berkeley
    Publishing Group, 1997.

Strand, R. D. *BioNutrition*. Rapid City, SD: Comprehensive Wellness
    Publishing, 1998.

Thurston-Temple, L., and B. Laughlin. *The Marriage of the Spirit*. Santa Fe,
    NM: CoreLight Publishing, 2000.

Weil, A. *Eating Well for Optimum Health*. New York: HarperCollins, 2000.

Weil, A. *Eight Weeks to Optimum Health*. New York: Fawcett Book Group,
    1998.

Whitaker, J. *Dr. Whitaker's Guide to Natural Healing*. Roseville, CA Prima
    Publishing, 1996.

Williams E., and I. Rosenberg. *Biomarkers*. New York: Simon and Schuster,
    1991.

Yoke, M., and L. Gladwin. *A Guide to Personal Fitness Training.
    Sherman Oaks, CA: Aerobics and Fitness Association of America,
    1997.*

Interested in Learning More About Optimum Health and Vitality?

You can receive a free one-year subscription of the *VITALITY CONNECTION* newsletter in an electronic format, containing the latest health and vitality news along with special offers, by contacting VitalityPress Publications via Email, facsimile, or mail. Please refer to the contact information provided below and include the following information in your request (all information is required):

Yes, I would like to receive a one-year subscription of the *VITALITY CONNECTION* newsletter for free!

Name (first and last) _____

Address _____

City, State, Zip _____

Email address _____

How did you obtain *The Vitality Connection?* _____

_____

Date of purchase _____

To learn more about the wellness workshops, personal wellness coaching, anti-aging treatments, and nutritional programs offered by the authors, contact:

VitalityPress Publications
111 Pacifica, Suite 250
Irvine, California 92618
USA
Phone: 949.770.0723
Fax: 949.380.7122
Email: inquiry@wanvitality.com